How to Succeed at Revalidation

How to Succeed at Revalidation

Peter Donnelly, MB BCH BAO, FRCPsych, BA(OU), FAcadMed, FHEA, FRCP(Ed), MMed, HonFAcadMed
Consultant Psychiatrist
Clinical Group Deputy Medical Director
Swansea Bay University Health Board
Swansea, UK

Katie Webb, BA (hons, BPS), MSc, PhD, CPsychol, FAcadMed
Lecturer in Evaluation and Standardisation
School of Medicine
Cardiff University
Cardiff, UK

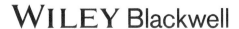

Registered Office(s)
John Wiley & Sons, Inc., 111 River Street, Hoboken, NJ 07030, USA
John Wiley & Sons Ltd, The Atrium, Southern Gate, Chichester, West Sussex, PO19 8SQ, UK

Editorial Office
9600 Garsington Road, Oxford, OX4 2DQ, UK

For details of our global editorial offices, customer services, and more information about Wiley products visit us at www.wiley.com.

Wiley also publishes its books in a variety of electronic formats and by print-on-demand. Some content that appears in standard print versions of this book may not be available in other formats.

Library of Congress Cataloging-in-Publication Data

Names: Donnelly, Peter, 1958– author. | Webb, Katie, 1974– author.
Title: How to succeed at revalidation / Peter Donnelly, Katie Webb.
Description: First edition. | Hoboken, NJ : Wiley, 2022. | Includes
    bibliographical references and index.
Identifiers: LCCN 2021021048 (print) | LCCN 2021021049 (ebook) | ISBN
    9781119650379 (paperback) | ISBN 9781119650362 (adobe pdf) | ISBN
    9781119650348 (epub)
Subjects: MESH: Credentialing–standards | Physicians–standards | Clinical
    Competence–standards | United Kingdom
Classification: LCC R834.5 (print) | LCC R834.5 (ebook) | NLM W 21 | DDC
    610.76–dc23
LC record available at https://lccn.loc.gov/2021021048
LC ebook record available at https://lccn.loc.gov/2021021049

Cover Design: Wiley
Cover Image: © TECHDESIGNWORK/Getty Images

Set in 9.5/12pt Minion by Straive, Pondicherry, India
Printed and bound by CPI Group (UK) Ltd, Croydon, CR0 4YY

C9781119650379_070921

Contents

Acknowledgments

Peter would like to thank all colleagues, in the NHS and across the wider health sector, whose views and opinions have helped shape this book. He would also like to thank his co-author Katie for her support.

Katie would like to thank her colleagues in Cardiff Medical School and in the NHS for their support at these challenging times. She would also like to thank her parents, Annie and Roger, for their continued support, as well as the patience and encouragement of Évie and Amélie.

Abbreviations

ACAT	Acute Care Assessment Tool
AD	Associate Dean
AoMRC	Academy of Medical Royal Colleges
ARCP	Annual Review of Competency Progression
BMA	British Medical Association
BRI	Bristol Royal Infirmary
CCT	Certificate of Completion of Training
CD	Clinical Director
CHI	Commission for Health Improvement
CMO	Chief Medical Officer
COPMeD	Conference of Postgraduate Medical Deans
CPD	Continuing Professional Development
CQC	Care Quality Commission
CRPS	Chronic Regional Pain Syndrome
CSP	Chartered Society of Physiotherapy
DB	Designated Body
DEN	Doctor's Educational Need
DISQ	Doctors Interpersonal Skills Questionnaire
DOPS	Direct Observation of Procedural Skills
ELA	Employer Liaison Adviser
GDC	General Dental Council
GIM	General Internal Medicine
GMC	General Medical Council
GMP	Good Medical Practice
GNM	Gross Negligence Manslaughter
GOC	General Optical Council
GP	General Practitioner
GPAQ	General Practice Assessment Questionnaire
GPAS	General Practice Assessment Survey
GPC	Generic Professional Capabilities
HEIW	Health Education and Improvement Wales

HPC	Health Professionals Council
ISQ	Interpersonal Skills Questionnaire
IT	Information Technology
JRCPTB	Joint Royal Colleges of Physicians Training Board
LGA	Local Government Association
MARS	Medical Appraisal and Revalidation System
MDT	Multi-Disciplinary Team
mini-CEX	Mini-Clinical Evaluation Exercise
MSF	Multi-Source Feedback
NCDA	National Cancer Diagnosis Audit
NELA	National Emergency Laparotomy Audit
NICE	National Institute for Health and Clinical Excellence
NMC	Nursing and Midwifery Council
NTN	National Training Number
PA	Physician Associate
PDP	Professional Development Plan
PEI	Patient Enablement Instrument
PREM	Patient-Reported Experience Measure
PROM	Patient-Reported Outcome Measure
PSQ	Patient Satisfaction Questionnaire
PUN	Patient's Unmet Need
QI	Quality Improvement
RCs	Royal Colleges
RCGP	Royal College of General Practitioners
RCP	Royal College of Physicians
RCPsych	Royal College of Psychiatrists
RCS	Royal College of Surgeons
RO	Responsible Officer
SAS	Staff and Associate Specialist
SEA	Significant Event Analysis
SI	Supporting Information
SLE	Supervised Learning Event
SOAR	Scotland Online Appraise Resource
SWOT	Strengths, Weaknesses, Opportunities, Threats
UK	United Kingdom
UKCC	United Kingdom Central Council for Nursing, Midwifery and Health Visiting
UKRPB	UK Revalidation Programme Board
VC	Video Consultation
WPBA	Workplace-Based Assessment

Chapter 1 **Introduction**

Working as a health care professional in the twenty-first century is both rewarding and challenging. Being a doctor is a complex role typically with a broad scope of practice, which includes not just one's clinical role but other responsibilities such as teaching, research and management. Whatever clinical area or specialty you are working in, there are increasing public expectations. Medical revalidation, introduced by the General Medical Council (GMC) in 2012, is an evaluation of a doctor's fitness to practice (GMC 2020).

What is this book about? This book reviews the background that led to the implementation of medical revalidation in the United Kingdom (UK). It also provides a comprehensive description of the current revalidation process for all doctors in the UK.

Who is this book for? This book is aimed at:

- All doctors in the UK who are subject to revalidation, including General Practitioners (GPs), Consultants, Staff and Associate Specialists (SASs), Locally Employed Doctors and Doctors in Training
- All doctors who are appraisers and or Responsible Officers
- All who are involved in postgraduate medical education and training
- All medical students and their tutors and lecturers.

Overview of the Book

This book explores the evolution of the regulatory processes in medicine and other health professionals from a UK and international perspective. The current UK regulatory framework is described, as well as the recent drivers for change. The book provides a step-by-step guide to the process of revalidation from the perspective of the appraisee, the appraiser, the Responsible Officer

How to Succeed at Revalidation, First Edition. Peter Donnelly and Katie Webb.
© 2022 John Wiley & Sons Ltd. Published 2022 by John Wiley & Sons Ltd.

and the employer. Examples of reflective writing are explored mapped to Good Medical Practice (GMP) and the Generic Professional Capabilities (GPCs). We then go on to explore the possible future for medical revalidation in the UK.

Background

The GMC considered the introduction of revalidation as far back as 1998. In 2010, the GMC together with the Chief Medical Officers (CMOs) from the four UK nations issued a joint Statement of Intent, explicitly defining the purpose of revalidation:

> *the purpose of revalidation is to assure patients and the public, employers and other health care professionals that licenced doctors are up to date and fit to practice*

> (Pearson 2017)

The process was eventually introduced in December 2012, but this change was not triggered by a single event but rather a cultural and systems shift in the UK and indeed across all health care systems globally. An increased expectation of the public, in part driven by increasingly better informed patients via the use of the internet and social media, and a number of high-profile malpractice cases have focused the attention of the public on the governance arrangements for health care professionals, including doctors. These events have included the scandals at the Bristol Royal Infirmary (Kennedy 2001), the issues at Alder Hey Children's Hospital (The Stationery Office 2001) and the Mid Staffordshire Report (Francis 2013).

As just one example, Francis (2013) in his final report into Mid Staffordshire discussed the use of appraisal to facilitate cultural change in NHS organizations, with a need for appraisal to be driven by feedback from patients and colleagues.

In the last 20–30 years, the models of care used to provide services to patients have been transformed, resulting in a greater emphasis on doctors working within multi-professional teams.

We are now also in the third medical revolution. The first was the public health revolution epitomized by the discovery that the 1854 cholera outbreak in London was as a result of contaminated water via the water pump on Broad Street, in the Soho area (now Broadwick Street), and not by airborne transmission. This finding led to the emergence of public health medicine.

The second has been the technological revolution over the last 50 years with investment in evidence-based medicine and a focus on quality of care, for example, Magnetic Resonance Imaging, coronary artery bypass graft surgery, joint replacements, chemotherapy, renal dialysis, to mention just a few.

The third medical revolution, triggered by the citizen and driven by knowledge and the internet, has led to digital health strategies delivering direct clinical care and supporting education training and ongoing professional development (Topol 2019).

The purpose of revalidation is to assure the public, patients, employers and other health care professionals that all licenced doctors are up to date and fit to practice.

The process of revalidation is underpinned by each doctor being actively engaged in annual appraisal. Appraisal should be supportive and developmental with a key element being reflection on the breadth of the doctor's professional practice with the desired outcome of improving the quality of care for patients. The reflection process should focus on events and learning and how they have applied that learning in practice (Kolb 1984).

All doctors in the UK are required to revalidate. There are two pathways: those working as GPs, Consultants and SAS doctors who do so through an annual appraisal process; and those doctors in training, in GMC-approved training programs who are subject to an Annual Review of Competency Progression (ARCP). This acts as an annual appraisal.

More recently, the GMC and other stakeholders recognized that, in achieving the UK certificate of completion of training (CCT), doctors in training should have to demonstrate an appropriate and mature professional identity, appropriate to their level of seniority. As a result, the GPCs, a set of common generic outcomes, were introduced across all postgraduate medical curricula (GMC 2017). There are currently 66 medical specialties and 32 sub-specialties in the UK and there has been significant variation across all of these curricula in terms of generic professional practice outcomes and expectations.

Challenges

Is medical revalidation fit for purpose? The UK is nearly through the second cycle of revalidation and it is clear there are still challenges in engagement, the quality of appraisal, and the process of ensuring a consistent approach (Pearson 2017). There remain a number of gaps and areas for improvement.

Moving forward there may be increasing pressure from society for an even more rigorous assessment of each individual doctor's level of knowledge and skill. Revalidation in the future is likely to require further changes to help meet the ever-evolving needs of the public and governments.

References

Francis, R. (2013). *Report of the Mid Staffordshire NHS Foundation Trust Public Inquiry (Report)*. London: The Stationery Office. https://www.gov.uk/government/publications/report-of-the-mid-staffordshire-nhs-foundation-trust-public-inquiry (accessed 5 May 2021).

General Medical Council (2017). *Generic professional capabilities framework*. Manchester: General Medical Council. https://www.gmc-uk.org/education/standards-guidance-and-curricula/standards-and-outcomes/generic-professional-capabilities-framework (accessed 5 May 2021).

General Medical Council (2020). *Guidance on supporting information for appraisal and revalidation*. Manchester: General Medical Council. https://www.gmc-uk.org/registration-and-licensing/managing-your-registration/revalidation/guidance-on-supporting-information-for-appraisal-and-revalidation (accessed 5 May 2021).

Kennedy, I. (2001). *The report of the public inquiry into children's heart surgery at the Bristol Royal Infirmary 1984–1995: Learning from Bristol*. The Bristol Royal Infirmary Inquiry. http://www.wales.nhs.uk/sites3/documents/441/The%20Kennedy%20Report.pdf (accessed 5 May 2021).

Kolb, D.A. (1984). *Experiential Learning: Experience as the Source of Learning and Development*. Englewood Cliffs, NJ: Prentice Hall.

Pearson, K. (2017). *Taking revalidation forward. Improving the process of relicensing for doctors*. Manchester: General Medical Council. https://www.gmc-uk.org/-/media/documents/Taking_revalidation_forward___Improving_the_process_of_relicensing_for_doctors.pdf_68683704.pdf (accessed 5 May 2021).

The Stationery Office (2001). *The Royal Liverpool Children's Inquiry Report*. London: The Stationery Office. https://www.gov.uk/government/publications/the-royal-liverpool-childrens-inquiry-report (accessed 5 May 2021).

Topol, E. (2019). *The Topol Review. Preparing the healthcare workforce to deliver the digital future. An independent report on behalf of the Secretary of State for Health and Social Care*. Health Education England. https://topol.hee.nhs.uk/ (accessed 5 May 2021).

Chapter 2 **Regulation in Health – A Brief History**

Introduction

In this chapter, we will explore the origins, evolution and development of regulation of the professions of nursing, physiotherapy and medicine. Whilst describing the development of these health care professions we will explore the historical development of the regulatory processes applying to these.

What is Regulation?

Before going on to explore regulation in a number of health professions, it is useful to consider briefly the development of regulation as a concept.

In general terms, regulation describes the rules that are set out in legislation and the processes used to monitor and enforce those rules. Regulation complements other government levers such as taxation and public spending in shaping society. In the business world the aim of regulation is to help in the delivery of better outcomes for the economy, society and the environment. In health care, the purpose of regulation is to ensure that all health professions are fit to practice and hence patient safety and public confidence is assured.

Regulation can have a significant impact on innovation. On the one hand it can stimulate innovative ideas, while on the other hand serve to hinder their implementation. As a result, regulation can either stimulate improvement and/or investment, or lead to a tick-box approach to regulatory compliance.

There are a number of subtypes of regulation:
- Arbitrary regulations – rules that mandate the use of one of several equally valid options (e.g. driving on the right- or left-hand side of the road)
- Good faith regulations – that aim to define a baseline of acceptable practice (e.g. food hygiene regulations for the hospitality industry)

How to Succeed at Revalidation, First Edition. Peter Donnelly and Katie Webb.
© 2022 John Wiley & Sons Ltd. Published 2022 by John Wiley & Sons Ltd.

- Goal conflict regulations – regulations that recognize a conflict between two parties and mandate for the greater good. These are typically conflicts between the individual versus wider society
- Process regulations – these determine how a task should be accomplished.

In addition, it is important to understand the characteristics of the regulator. In peer-regulation the community regulates itself, a form of self-regulation. Unilateral or flat regulation is when regulations are imposed by the body with the power to do so. Statutory regulation is where the authority to define the rules is delegated to an independent third party body. This is the current position with health regulation in the UK whereby the Government delegates power to regulatory bodies such as the General Medical Council (GMC) or the General Dental Council (GDC).

In general, any forward-thinking society would wish for regulation that supports and stimulates innovation, which in turn benefits citizens and the economy. In addition, optimal regulation is one that protects members of the public but does not hinder innovation and/or have unintended negative consequences. Across all sectors there is a need for regulators to evolve to keep pace with the rapid changes in society, and with the need to maintain the balance of safety and security versus innovation that improves the lives of its citizens.

Regulation in Health Professions

Professionalism and Society

In early history, occupations began to evolve and move into what would now be considered a profession. The key milestones marking this transition from simple activity to a profession include full-time occupation, establishment of training schools or universities, codes of ethics and regulation, licensing legislation and colleague control. Another key component in this transition to a profession was the balance between a level of autonomy of work and the regulatory requirements. Larson added to the characteristics above with the addition of high standards of professional and intellectual excellence, as well as referring to professions as "exclusive elite groups" (Larson 1978, p. 20).

The three original occupations of law, the clergy and medicine arose through the medieval universities of Europe. By the turn of the nineteenth century, with occupation specialization, different bodies claimed and achieved professional status including nursing and teaching.

The concept of medical professionalism probably dates back to the late medieval times when doctors organized a professional guild (Sox 2002). At that point medical professionalism was viewed as the art of practicing medicine to a certain set of standards that were set by the profession itself, essentially self-regulation. This has evolved and responded to societal and political changes. The professions addressed a range of societal issues and in return society afforded these professions a number of privileges, including monopoly status, the authority to decide who could enter the profession and the ability to influence government policy.

In essence there was an implied social contract (Cruess et al. 2010) where there was an acceptance of the balance between altruism and self-regulation. Although early definitions of the medical profession have been doctor-centered, there has been a shift recognized by regulatory bodies toward a position of medical professionalism as being a social construct, a social contract between doctors and society (Cruess and Cruess 2008).

The social contract is now recognized as a tripartite agreement involving three interconnected societal elements:
1 The government, employers, and health care managers
2 Patients, patient groups and the general population
3 The medical profession and its professional bodies.

Each of these groups has its own responsibilities and roles in fulfilling its side of the contract. There is recognition from certain sections of the medical profession that the social contract is a dynamic entity that is ever-changing in the context of rising systematic pressures and societal expectations. There are many factors that impact upon the contract, including the regulators, social media, print and broadcast media, and professional organizations (Cruess and Cruess 2011).

Recognizing the evolving position, in 2015 Jeremy Hunt, the then Health Secretary, called for a new social contract between the public, health and care services. In a speech to the Local Government Association (LGA) annual conference in Harrogate, Mr. Hunt urged the public to take more personal responsibility:
- for looking after the elderly
- for their own health
- in using finite NHS resources.

He argued that, while integration of health and social care is vital to delivering the highest standards of health and care, personal responsibility needs to sit alongside system accountability (Hunt 2015).

There is a further element to the evolution of health roles. It has been argued that there has been a significant blurring between the roles of health professions. There are arguments for and against this development. Although roles have evolved and are constantly changing, there is a current strategic position in the UK from governments and the relevant statutory education and training bodies to actively upskill non-medical professions and develop new roles such as the Physician Associate (PA). There are possible risks with this strategy, and some argue that these developments have been accelerated to reduce costs and that there is a risk the system now expects some professions to work beyond their competency ceiling (Oxtoby 2009).

Self-Regulation

While we will explore self-regulation in relation to medicine in greater detail later in the chapter, the concept of self-regulation has been defined as a contract between the profession and the public (represented by the State). As a part of the contract, the profession promises that all members of the public will be served by good doctors and protected from bad ones. In turn the public, via the State, gives the profession a high level of autonomy over its own affairs. There are arguments for and against self-regulation. The first in favor of self-regulation is that medicine is so complex that doctors themselves are best placed to define standards that differentiate between good and unacceptable practice. The second argument is that if doctors as a body have a sense of ownership of these standards, then they are more likely to adhere to them. The argument goes that such a model of self-regulation, if balanced with processes to ensure the public has a loud voice, is the best to achieve the desired outcome – a safer service for patients.

Professional regulation has two key elements. The first is at the level of the individual doctor. This requires individual doctors to exercise self-discipline. This requirement is of paramount importance considering the clinical scenarios facing most doctors on a daily basis where they have to make decisions, with patients, based on less than optimal evidence (Bate et al. 2012).

The second element lies at the collective level where the profession as a whole is required to ensure that current practice, in general, is in line with the accepted standards in operation at that time. These standards are by their nature changing frequently. For example, the legal framework underpinning the process of obtaining consent in the UK changed significantly after the Montgomery case in 2015 (Chan et al. 2017).

In order to set the context for the current regulatory framework in medicine, explored in Chapter 3, the history of the evolution of regulation for nursing, physiotherapy, and medicine will be briefly explored here. The evolution of regulation of each of these professions are intrinsically linked as the social and political pressures and levers have been similar for each.

The Nursing Profession

The term "nurse" is derived from the Italian word, *nutrire*, meaning to feed, nourish or suckle a baby. The earliest written records of nurses are from the Roman Empire.

In ancient Greece, approximately between 460 and 375 BCE, Hippocrates realized that human disease was based on biology and not supernatural causes. He developed the concept of physical observations and reporting on the holistic health of the patient. He is famous for writing the Hippocratic Oath, which was a pledge that all doctors had to take. Although in recent years the Oath has fallen out of favor, a survey of all medical schools in the UK found that 70% of those responded still used a version of the oath (Green 2017).

Throughout the early middle ages, health care and therefore nursing in England was set within and controlled by the churches, mainly the Roman Catholic Church.

The Reformation, a movement across Europe, began in about 1517 driven in part by Martin Luther, and posed serious political and religious challenges to the Roman Catholic Church and specifically to the authority of the Pope. In England, the Reformation under the reign of Henry VIII led to the Church of England breaking away from Catholicism. This then led to the dissolution of monasteries between 1536 and 1541, and the shutting down of the associated hospitals and infirmary buildings. This has come to be known as the "Dark Age of Nursing" as the English Reformation resulted in many hospitals being closed down. The larger hospitals in London such as St Thomas' and St Bartholomew's, although at risk through the Reformation, were able to survive with their management taken over by the City of London. Henry VIII's only son Edward VI ordered charters for the continued use of these organizations and institutions as hospitals.

Throughout this period there was no, or very little, formal training for those who considered nursing as a job. Nurses were seen as subordinates, servants and individuals who were given nursing jobs instead of, for example, a prison sentence. Nurses were generally disregarded by society and other health professions.

The professional era for nursing began with the establishment of the first training school for nursing in Kaiserswerth, Germany, in 1836. The school was founded by the Lutheran Order of Deaconesses for the purpose of providing high-quality nursing training to the Deaconesses.

The Anglican Nursing Sisterhood of St John's had developed a Nurse Teaching School in London in approximately 1848. As well as providing successful clinical training, the nursing school supported the individual's spiritual calling with a real emphasis on the all-important Christian duty expected in this Victorian era.

In 1856 the Sisterhood took over nursing at King's College Hospital, London, and then in 1866 took over responsibility for nursing at Charing Cross Hospital. It was also known as the Training Institution for Nurses for Hospitals, Families and the Sick Poor. At that stage nurse training was a combination of clinical training and religious education, highlighting the continuing control the church had on health.

It is argued that the world's first non-religious nurse training school, "La Source" was established in Lausanne in Switzerland. It was founded in 1859, a year before the Nightingale Training School in St Thomas' opened.

Florence Nightingale, considered by most to be the founder of modern nursing, studied at Kaiserswerth and on returning to England she became superintendent for the Institution for the Care of Sick Gentlewomen in Distressed Circumstances in London.

The Crimean War began in 1853, and news reports described deplorable conditions and a lack of medical or nursing care for injured British troops. Nightingale was asked by the British Government to go to the Crimea and organize better care for the troops. Accompanied by a number of nurses, Nightingale found the troops experiencing horrifying conditions. She set about transforming the general conditions of the soldiers, and the main impact was as a result of improvements in sanitation and hygiene, leading to improved clinical outcomes.

Following her experiences in the Crimea, Nightingale returned to London and in 1860 established the first secular nurse training school in the UK at St Thomas' Hospital London – the Nightingale Training School. Nightingale's new training system was described as ground-breaking at that time. It was noted that the Nightingale Training School, while being the second non-religious nursing school, adopted the "sisterhood" approach to training and instigated the ward system. Nightingale's initiative was opposed by many physicians at the time who argued that nurses needed only minimal training, enough to provide cleanliness, poultice-making and attending to patients' personal needs (Kalish and Kalish 1995). History records that Nightingale set up the foundations for non-secular training of women of "good character" from all backgrounds. A further unique element of Nightingale's approach was the recognition of science as the essential basis for nursing care.

In 1849 Pastor Fliedner, who was the driving force in setting up Kaiserswerth, established the first Protestant hospital in America. The trained Deaconesses who travelled with him started the first formal nurse training program in the Pittsburgh Infirmary, Pennsylvania, which still exists today as the Passavant Hospital.

When state registration of doctors in the UK began in 1858, there was also a call for registration of trained nurses. In 1887, the British Nurses Association was created and received the Royal Charter in 1892, becoming the Royal British Nurses Association (RBNA). Princess Helena, the daughter of Queen Victoria, was president of the RBNA and was keen to enhance the training and status of nursing. The RBNA was in favor of registration as a means to ensure and enhance the professional status of trained nurses.

The First World War acted as a catalyst for the regulation of nursing. During the war the role of women, in general, in British society changed. The number of women in paid employment almost doubled from 1914 to 1918, and women were working in occupations they would previously have been excluded from, including heavy industry such as shipbuilding. At the end of the war over eight million women were granted the right to vote for the first time, and the Eligibility of Women Act 1918 allowed some women to be elected as Members of Parliament.

In addition, nursing increasingly contributed to the war effort. There was a significant increase in the number of nurses in the military, and at the end of the war there were over 10 000 nurses working in the Queen Alexandra's Imperial Military Nursing service. This coincided with the establishment of the College of Nursing in 1916. In 1919 a Private Members Bill was passed, the Nurse Registration Act, providing the legislation for formal nurse registration. This resulted in the establishment of the General Nurse Council for England and Wales.

Throughout the 1920s to the 1970s the nursing profession fought for further recognition, with a focus on pay and conditions, quality of training, and status of role in the NHS, amongst many other issues.

In 1979, further legislative changes created the United Kingdom Central Council (UKCC) for Nursing, Midwifery and Health Visiting, a new regulatory body being formally established in 1983. The purpose of the UKCC was to maintain a register of all UK nurses, midwifes and health visitors, produce guidance for registrants, and handle any complaints. In 2002 the UKCC became the Nursing and Midwifery Council (NMC) that exists today. The stated purpose of the NMC is (NMC 2020):

> We maintain the register of nurses and midwifes who meet the requirements for registration in the UK, and nursing associates who meet the requirements for registration in England.
>
> We set the requirements for the professional education that supports people to develop the knowledge, skills and behaviour required for entry to, or annotation on, our register.
>
> We shape the practice of the professional on our register by developing and promoting standards including our Code, and we promote lifelong learning through revalidation.
>
> Where serious concerns are raised about a nurse, midwife or nurse associate's fitness to practice, we can investigate and, if needed, take action.

The NMC has published a detailed code of practice, "the Code," which forms the reference point for revalidation of nurses. Table 2.1 shows the requirements for and examples of the supporting evidence for each registrant over a three-year cycle in order to revalidate.

Table 2.1 Revalidation: requirements of a nurse and examples of supporting evidence.

Requirements over a three-year cycle	Supporting evidence
450 hours of practice for each registration (if dual registration requires 900 hours)	Record of practice hours Scope of practice Details of the work setting
35 hours of continuing professional development (of which 20 hours must be participatory)	Details of the CPD recorded including: The CPD method used (e.g. online, self-learning) Each CPD session mapped to the code
Five pieces of practice-related feedback	Notes on the feedback Details of how feedback used to improve practice
Five written reflective accounts	Written reflection on CPD/feedback or an event/experience Describe relevance to the code
Reflective discussion	Record of a reflective discussion NMC number of the person
Health and character	Self-declaration of health and character
Professional indemnity	Evidence of appropriate professional indemnity
Confirmation	Following face-to-face or video meeting, a record of the conversation with an appropriate "confirmer," e.g. line manager or a GP

As we will see in later chapters, this process shares many of the elements of the current revalidation requirements for doctors.

Physiotherapy

The origins of the profession of physiotherapy are thought to date back as far as Hippocrates, the ancient Greek physician who lived during Greece's Classical period (c. 400 BCE). He advocated the use of physical therapies to treat a number of ailments.

The profession began in earnest in 1813 when Per Henrik Ling founded the Royal Central Institute of Gymnastics in Sweden. Ling recognized the benefits of massage, physical manipulation and exercise, not just in treating ailments but in the prevention of disease.

The Society of Trained Masseuses was established in 1894 in order to protect the profession from falling into disrepute as a result of a number of newspaper articles. The society's emphasis was on the medical model for massage training and high academic standards. By 1900 the Society progressed to obtaining the legal status of a professional organization and became the

Incorporated Society of Trained Masseuses. This helped to improve the public's perception of the profession.

The society was granted the Royal Charter in 1920 and joined with the Institute of Massage and Remedial Gymnastics. The society and the profession grew and in 1944 it became the Charted Society of Physiotherapy (CSP), its name to this day.

Then in 1976, the society was also recognized as an independent trade union. It was not until 1977 that the Department of Health recognized professional autonomy for physiotherapists, and the following year a change in law allowed direct referrals to physiotherapists without the need for a medical referral.

In 1992 the physiotherapy profession became an all-graduate entry profession. The Health Professionals Council (HPC) replaced the Council for the Professions Supplementary to Medicine (CPSM), and physiotherapy came under the regulation of the HPC in 2003. This established legal protection for the titles of "Physiotherapist" and "Physical Therapist."

Medicine

The history of the physician dates back as far as the history of mankind. In 3500 BCE the Egyptians were documenting the "medicine" of the time. At that time the practice of medicine was intertwined with religious and magical beliefs, customs and practice.

Around 800 BCE, Homer talked of drugs being administered along with magical spells. A range of minerals, vegetation and animal parts were used to make up the drugs. In many cultures those who dealt with diseases were priests or holy men.

One of the earliest recorded calls for regulation in the UK was in 1421. Physicians presented a petition to parliament canvassing to ensure that anyone practicing as a physician should have appropriate qualifications.

In 1511 a statute placed the regulation of physicians in the hands of the Bishops in England on the basis that the clerics were, in general, the best educated of any social group in the population. So, even in the sixteenth century, medicine and the practice of religion remained closely aligned.

Before the Medical Act of 1858 the organizational structure of medicine in the UK was close to a state of chaos. By the early 1800s there were 19 different licensing bodies in the UK with a whole range of rules governing recognition of physicians. Medical training varied from basic apprenticeship in an apothecary shop to classical university education with a degree in medicine.

There were a wide number of "quacks" and drug peddlers practicing with no legal sanction against them. On the other hand a physician based in

London could be disciplined by the Royal College of Physicians (RCP) for preparing and selling a prescription.

To understand the nature and development of this near-chaotic situation, it is important to understand the historical developments. One key issue was the separation of "medical men" into three orders: Physicians, Surgeons and Apothecaries. These orders fell under the Royal College of Physicians (RCP), the Royal College of Surgeons (RCS) and the Society of Apothecaries respectively. These three orders of medical practice very much reflected the social divisions of society at that time. Each group had their own legal rights and duties, traditional and historical privileges, exclusivity of membership and functions, and monopoly on activities.

Physicians

The oldest medical organization in the UK was the RCP in London who received the Royal Charter in 1518. It is important to understand that at that time, the scope of practice of a Physician is most similar to what we would now consider to be exclusively internal medicine. Fellows of the Royal College had to practice within strict limitations and, for example, they could not belong to any other medical organization. Neither could they practice surgery or act as an apothecary. This meant Fellows were prohibited from making or selling medicines even to their own patients. There was a requirement for a Fellow of the Royal College to act only as a pure physician examining, diagnosing and prescribing medication which was then dispensed by the apothecary. The rules were such that if a Physician decided to start practicing surgery or dispensing drugs, he had to resign his Fellowship or face expulsion. The RCP fought hard to maintain the distinction between Physicians and other orders of practitioners such as surgeons and apothecaries.

What really set the RCP apart from the other two orders of medical practitioners was that they restricted the offering of Fellowship to those individuals with university degrees. However, in terms of scale, the number of physicians was small. In 1800 there were a total of 179 Fellows in England; by 1847 this number had grown to 683. Of these, 76 resided in London, showing that over this period of time the influence of the RCP, which essentially started life as a London-only organization, had spread to medical practitioners across England. Having said that, the RCP represented less than 5% of all medical practitioners in England by the mid-1800s.

Surgeons

With regard to surgery it was clear that surgeons had operated as an ancient medical art as far back as the physician. The surgeon performed operations, set broken bones, treated accident cases, and much of the surgeon's work demanded high levels of hand–eye coordination, dexterity, speed, decision-making, as well as expertise. It was considered a form of skilled manual labor, and the eighteenth century phrase "The Craft of Surgery" still resonates today in the narrative of surgery as a craft specialty.

Since the middle ages, surgeons in the London area had been organized as a guild. Guilds were associations of merchants or artisans with mutual interests. They were organizations that operated like a combination of a trade union and a professional body. It was only in 1540 that they joined with the barbers to form the Barber–Surgeons Company of the City of London. This relationship lasted until 1745 when the surgeons established a separate city company. In 1800 the surgeons received their Charter as the Royal College of Surgeons of London, and then in 1843 they were made the Royal College of Surgeons (RCS) of England, with the establishment of Membership (MRCS) and Fellowship (FRCS) which remains today.

An important distinction between physicians and surgeons at that point was that surgeons were not university educated. They learned their skills through apprenticeships and by practical training, and not in any way theoretical or university-based.

The RCS was much larger than the RCP. By the mid-nineteenth century there were over 8000 practitioners with a surgical license, but only 300 of these were Fellows of the College. The FRCS was not an exclusively London license, and those who held it could practice in all parts of England.

In order to make a living, most members of the RCS also began to prescribe and dispense drugs, and in order to qualify themselves for this they took on a second qualification from the Apothecary Society.

Apothecaries

Before 1617, Apothecaries had been a part of the Grocers' Company of the City of London. It was in that year they obtained a Royal Charter as the Society of Apothecaries. Their charter stipulated that they were responsible for the supply, compounding and sale of drugs in London, and they were distinguished from physicians and surgeons by not being called medical practitioners but "Druggists."

In 1815 the Apothecaries Act legitimized the practice of medicine by apothecaries and authorized the Society of Apothecaries to grant a Licence of the Society of Apothecaries (LSA) Medical Practice in England. Similar to surgeons, apothecaries were trained by an apprenticeship model and not via a university-based degree.

The LSA became an increasingly popular qualification amongst medical practitioners, with increasing numbers of physicians granted licenses, allowing them to dispense drugs to their own patients.

So, in the early nineteenth century the landscape of the medical profession in England consisted of three discrete and separately organized professions. These professions were legally defined status groups whose activities were defined by a charter devised by their relevant Royal College or Society. The three professions were ranked in a hierarchical basis with physicians above surgeons, who were perceived as superior to apothecaries. This reflected the explicit class and hierarchical system in society at that time.

Therefore, set against this background, when any reforms into medical regulations were discussed or considered, this typically triggered significant resistance amongst these separate organizations.

Outside of the elite group within the Royal Colleges, day-to-day medical practice started to coalesce among the three orders of practitioners. So, on a day-to-day basis medical care was less compartmentalized. For example, after the Apothecaries Act 1815, physicians who engaged in prescribing and dispensing drugs were required to take the LSA, irrespective of whatever other license they held. For members of the RCS, the LSA was not a legal requirement to undertake surgical practice, but it became accepted that by 1830s that surgical practitioners also held this qualification.

Structures on the ground began to change as well. It was really in the first 30 years of the nineteenth century that the term General Practitioner (GP) started to emerge, and this term referred to those who practiced medicine and surgery, whether they were licensed by their respective colleges or not.

Further evidence of the divergence away from the central elitist colleges based in London was the organic development of a wide range of supportive structures around the profession. Societies devoted to medical science, social clubs, medical book clubs and a range of medical and interest groups began to flourish. The politics evolved so that over time the majority of practitioners, whether surgical, medical or purely apothecaries, felt distant and isolated from central London and felt that their needs and requirements were not being met.

Although the passing of the Apothecaries Act was hailed as the beginning of medical reform, there were a number of unintended consequences, one of which was the merging of the identity of roles of the surgeon and the apothecary. Thus the act accelerated the process of breaking down distinctions between surgeons and apothecaries, and hence what had become in general, accepted practice on a day-to-day basis was enshrined in law.

This brief insight to the early nineteenth century medical world gives a sense of some of the structural and political resistances to change at that time. Despite the Medical Act of 1858, the training of doctors remained variable in quality throughout the 1800s (Peterson 1978).

One significant initiative, as a result of the Medical Act 1858, was the establishment of the forerunner to the GMC, called then the General Council of Medical Education and Registration of the UK. This body was responsible for registration and medical education across the UK.

The Medical Act 1950 established the GMC as it exists today. There remained, however, concerns with regard to the level of assurance and scrutiny. The Merrison Report (Secretary of State for Social Services 1975) made a number of recommendations including a restructuring of the disciplinary processes, particularly for doctors with mental health problems, and led to the development of greater specialization and GP registration. This in turn led to the new Medical Act in 1978. The more recent history of the evolution of medical regulation is covered in Chapter 3.

Current Health Regulators in the UK

The brief histories of three health professions explored above demonstrate an evolving picture in the UK. The professions' view of the appropriate level of regulation has varied across centuries, and the role and influence of the public has changed immeasurably.

A consultation by the UK government (Department of Health 2017) recognized that while there was a large number of health and social care regulators, there was an inconsistency in approach to regulation and in particular to how fitness-to-practice issues are handled. The number of regulatory bodies remains an issue yet to be resolved. Any future proposals to change by amalgamating bodies will be subject to further consultation. One might argue consulting that includes the bodies is not likely to provide a definitive answer.

Table 2.2 demonstrates the wide range of regulators, the profession each regulates, and the number of registrants involved.

Chapter Summary

The origins of health care and hence health professions date back to the beginning of *Homo sapiens*. There are a number of common threads in the evolution of all health care professions with early beginnings under the auspices of physicians, underpinned by faith, religion, and magic. With medicine, in its most general definition, as the profession evolved any external regulation was essentially non-existent. The profession fought for the continuation of self-regulation and the luxury of the autonomy that afforded its members. There was the struggle against regulation and licensing from the clergy. Then with increasing expectations from the public (that the profession was there to serve the community), successive governments moved

Table 2.2 The UK regulators and the number of registrants (as of 2017/18).

Regulatory body	Professions covered	Number of registrants 2017/18
General Chiropractic Council (GCC)	Chiropractors	3255
General Dental Council (GDC)	Dentists Dental technicians Dental nurses Dental hygienists Dental therapists Orthodontic therapists	101 128
General Medical Council (GMC)	Medical practitioners	281 018
General Optical Council (GOC)	Optometrists Dispensing opticians Student optometrists Student dispensing opticians Optical businesses	30 097
General Osteopathic Council (GOsC)	Osteopaths	5239
General Pharmaceutical Council (GPhC)	Pharmacists Pharmacy technicians Pharmacy business premises	78 625 pharmacy professionals 14 348 pharmacy businesses
Health and Care Professions Council (HCPC)	Art therapist Biomedical scientists Chiropodists/podiatrists Clinical scientists Dieticians Hearing aid dispensers Occupational therapists Operating department practitioners Orthoptists Paramedics Physiotherapists Practitioner psychologists Prosthetists/orthotists Radiographers Social workers (England only) Speech and language therapists	361 061
Nursing and Midwifery Council (NMC)	Nurses Midwives Nursing Associates	690 773
Pharmaceutical Society of Northern Ireland (PSNI)	Pharmacists (NI) Pharmacy premises (NI)	2479 pharmacists 548 pharmacies
Social Care Wales (SCW)	Social workers (Wales)	TBC

more and more to legislative frameworks whereby regulation and licensing sat with bodies independent of the professions.

The three examples, nursing, physiotherapy, and medicine, then evolved, and with the advent of science, statistics, modern techniques and technology became well defined, but with continuing overlaps in skill and competencies such as the ability to prescribe medicines. The scope and hence status of all health professions is constantly evolving. A number of new professions in the sector (with Physician Associates as an example) has led to further blurring of professional boundaries.

It could be argued that recent consultation and the agreed recommendation does move health regulation further along the continuum from entirely self-regulated with no oversight, as was the case circa 50 years ago (Neighbour 2005), to a position of more rigorous governance where the voice and needs of the "public" play a bigger part.

If one reflects on the history of health professionals, clear silos existed in the 1700s, and although the origins can be traced back in history, they are very much alive today (McCarthney 2016).

References

Bate, L., Hutchinson, A., Underhill, J. et al. (2012). How clinical decisions are made. *British Journal of Clinical Pharmacology* **74** (4): 614–620.

Chan, S.W., Tulloch, E., Cooper, E.S. et al. (2017). Montgomery and informed consent: where are we now? *British Medical Journal* **357**: j2224. https://doi.org/10.1136/bmj.j2224.

Cruess, R.L. and Cruess, S.R. (2008). Expectations and obligations: professionalism and medicine's social contract with society. *Perspectives in Biology and Medicine* **51**: 579–598.

Cruess, S.R. and Cruess, R.L. (2011). Medicine's social contract with society. In: *Psychiatry's Contract with Society* (eds. D. Bhugra, A. Malik and G. Ikkos), 123–146. Oxford: OUP.

Cruess, S.R., Cruess, R.L., and Steinert, Y. (2010). Linking the teaching of professionalism to the social contract: a call for cultural humility. *Medical Teacher* **31**: 357–360.

Department of Health (2017). *Promoting professionalism, reforming regulation. A paper for consultation*. Department of Health. https://www.gov.uk/government/consultations/promoting-professionalism-reforming-regulation (accessed 6 May 2021).

Green, B. (2017). Use of the Hippocratic or other professional oaths in UK medical schools in 2017: practice, perception of benefit and principlism. *BMC Research Notes* **10**: 777. http://doi.org/10.1186/s13104-017-3114-7.

Hunt, J. (2015). New social contract between the public, health and care services. https://www.gov.uk/government/news/new-social-contract-between-the-public-health-and-care-services (accessed 6 May 2021).

Kalisch, P.A. and Kalisch, B.J. (1995). *American Nursing: A History*. Philadelphia, PA: Lippincott, Williams and Wilkins.

Larson, A.S. (1978). *The Rise of Professionalism: A Sociological Analysis*. Berkeley, CA: University of California Press.

McCarthney, M. (2016). Breaking down the silos walls. *British Medical Journal* https://doi.org/10.1136/bmj.i5199.

Neighbour, R. (2005). Rotten apples. *British Journal of General Practice* **55**: 241.

Nursing and Midwifery Council (2020). *About us*. https://nmc.org.uk/about-us (accessed 6 May 2021).

Oxtoby, K. (2009). Professional roles are blurring. *British Medical Journal* **338**: a3163. (accessed 1 February 2021).

Peterson, M.J. (1978). *The Medical Profession in Mid-Victorian*. London: University of California Press.

Secretary of State for Social Services (1975). *Report of the Committee of Inquiry into the Regulation of the Medical Profession*. Chairman Dr A.W. Merrison. Cmnd 6018. London: HMSO.

Sox, H. (2002). Medical professionalism project: medical professionalism in the new millennium – a physician's charter. *Annals of Internal Medicine* **136**: 243–246.

Chapter 3 **A History of the Current Framework**

Introduction

It is important to reflect on the steps that led to the current regulatory framework for medical revalidation, as this history may shine a light on the future of this process.

As we have seen in the previous chapter, throughout the early twentieth century there were no significant changes to the General Medical Council (GMC) and its role. A series of events and societal changes occurred that started to set the conditions for acceleration of change to the regulation of doctors.

As discussed in Chapter 2, medical practitioners were in three camps or tribes. The first was the Physician, a member of the Royal College of Physicians (RCP), and mainly from the higher social class. They generally administered to the wealthy and the aristocracy. The Surgeons on the other hand were mainly from the lower classes, until they separated from the Barbers, and then their status began to increase. The third group, the Apothecaries, were perceived as the lowest in the order.

From about the 1850s an important process emerged that led to a significant division of labor that still exists and remains a key driver for change and also a major constraint. The accepted process was that General Practitioners (GPs) retained the sole right of referral into hospital-based specialists. This process led to a division of labor and responsibility between GPs and those doctors who were hospital-based. This was a major factor in driving the increasing specialism in the delivery of care in hospitals. The hospital specialist provided treatment only when patients were in hospital. Also, specialists could not see patients directly but had to wait until they were referred by

How to Succeed at Revalidation, First Edition. Peter Donnelly and Katie Webb.
© 2022 John Wiley & Sons Ltd. Published 2022 by John Wiley & Sons Ltd.

the GP. Hence the GP consulted the hospital doctor, leading to the term "the consultant."

Those consultants based in hospitals started to focus more and more on sub-specialization and research. The GP on the other hand only required a basic medical degree to practice. The average GP would have undertook some surgery, delivered babies and lived within the communities they served: the "family doctor."

The Establishment of the National Health Service

The establishment of the NHS in 1948 by Aneurin Bevan, the then Health Secretary, had far-reaching consequences. For the first time, hospitals, doctors, nurses, pharmacists, opticians, and dentists were brought together under one umbrella organization to provide services that were free for all at the point of delivery.

An extract from a leaflet sent to all households in February 1948 reads:

> **Your new National Health Service begins on 5th July. What is it? How do you get it?**
>
> *It will provide you with all medical, dental and nursing care. Everyone – rich or poor, man, woman or child – can use it or any part of it. There are no charges, except for a few special items. There are no insurance qualifications. But it is not a "charity". You are all paying for it, mainly as tax payers, and it will relieve your money worries in time of illness.*
>
> (Society of Health 1980)

The NHS was built around the existing tribal processes and vested interest of the consultants and the GPs. The consultants were now salaried by the NHS, and GPs were self-employed, independent contractors. It was recognized from the outset that the NHS was under-funded and it could be argued that there developed a tacit agreement between successive governments and the profession that the GPs would effectively control referrals into hospital. This placed GPs as the "formal" gatekeepers for referrals and hence a controlling mechanism for costs. This cost-controlling mechanism was recognized and supported by successive governments. The political and societal price was to continue to allow the medical profession a high level of autonomy and hence continuance of self-regulation that the profession had enjoyed for centuries.

Within hospital-based services there evolved a picture of increasing sub-specialization, a hierarchical career structure, and a closed system of financial remuneration via the merit awards that Bevan had introduced himself.

As a result of all of these factors, consultant posts were highly sought after and highly competitive.

In contrast, in General Practice there was a lack of professional standards, with wide variation in the quality of the service patients could expect to receive. A report on GPs in the United Kingdom (Collings 1950) acted as a catalyst for the establishment of the Royal College of General Practitioners (RCGP) in 1952.

GPs still wanted the status of independent contractor and voted for a capitation fee, a basic fee per head of population served by each practice. This issue and insufficient investment in GP led to unhappiness. The British Medical Association (BMA), which had been set up in 1832 as the Provincial Medical and Surgical Association with the initial purpose as a vehicle to share scientific knowledge, becoming an independent trade union 1971, canvassed for a charter (British Medical Association 1965). This laid the foundations for the team-based primary care service that we recognize today.

This issue of a lack of agreed standards for GPs began to be addressed when the RCGP introduced a membership examination in 1965, the MRCGP, to test skills and competencies. The training needed to meet the examination requirements was voluntary and remained so until 1982. Over the ensuing years the RCGP and BMA fought over this issue, as the BMA wanted to ensure that any of its members who could not pass the examination could still earn a living as a GP. This protective approach by the BMA was not challenged by successive governments, who were content with the status quo.

Over this period of time, the role of the GMC was essentially passive and reactive to events. The main players were GPs, the consultant body, the BMA, and the established and emerging colleges. New Royal Colleges (RCs) were emerging, such as the RCs of Pathology in 1962 and Emergency Medicine in 1967. These organizations began to exercise their authority and also reacted to what they perceived to be the GMC's London-centric focus.

The Royal Commission on Medical Education (1965–1968)

Throughout the 1960s, the landscape of medicine was changing rapidly. Junior doctors were increasingly vocal about their conditions of employment, particularly the long hours and lack of supervision from senior colleagues.

These pressures and others triggered a Royal Commission on Medical Education (1965–1968) that led to further changes in both undergraduate (referred to as basic medical education) and postgraduate training. The commission produced a range of recommendations outlined below.

In undergraduate medical education, the first three years were to include studies in the preclinical sciences leading to a basic degree. After this, students were to undergo a further two years of clinical medicine and then be eligible to graduate. Following graduation, each would undertake a pre-registration intern year, after which they had the option of applying for specialized and vocational training. The first three years of post-intern training were to be general training and the last two years more specialized. It was recommended that there should be an overlap between each of the specialties to allow more flexibility in career pathways. This inflexibility in the training programs remains a key issue today (GMC 2019).

It was recommended that throughout the first three years of training each doctor would be regularly assessed, and following a final assessment would be issued with a Certificate approved by a new body, the Central Council for Postgraduate Medical Education and Training in Great Britain. Those doctors obtaining a high grade in this certificate would be eligible to enter a further two years of accelerated training to then be eligible for a consultant post.

The Royal Commission focused attention on improving the status and the attractiveness of general practice, but its recommendations did little to achieve this aim. For example, the Commission failed to recommend that GP posts were equivalent to consultants, but rather equated them to the generalist level obtained by doctors after just three years of post-intern training.

The Profession's Relationship with the GMC

In the early 1970s the profession was increasingly challenging the GMC. There were a number of triggers for this. The operating costs of the GMC were rising. The GMC did not have appropriate systems to support underperforming doctors, and the significant number of overseas doctors now recruited into supporting the NHS were not being dealt with. The GMC Council was lobbying Parliament to place specialist training under its control. This approach was resisted strongly by the Royal Colleges, and conflict between the Colleges and the GMC grew. One example of this growing tension was the lack of support from the GMC for the RCGP in its attempt to tackle poor practice in GPs.

These and other conflicts brought individual doctors, Royal Colleges and the BMA in direct conflict with the GMC. The focal point came in 1969 when the GMC proposed the introduction of an annual retention fee for all doctors, in order to solve their financial problems. Prior to that, there was a single fee for initial registration. There was outrage amongst the medical profession. As a result, the GMC and the BMA were at loggerheads over this issue from 1970 to 1972. The central issue was not the fee per se, but the perception that doctors and GPs in particular were not being represented in, or by, the GMC. The issue came to a crisis point in 1972 when the GMC Council voted to remove any doctor from the register if they had not paid the annual fee. Most doctors refused to pay the new fee and as a consequence, faced with the risk of thousands of doctors technically struck off for not paying, the government of the day intervened and appointed the Merrison Committee of Inquiry (Secretary of State for Social Services 1975). The terms of reference were:

> . . .to consider what changes need to be made in the existing provisions for the regulation of the medical profession; what functions should be assigned to the body charged with the responsibility for its regulation and how that body should be constituted to enable it to discharge its functions most effectively; and to make recommendation.
>
> (Irvine 2003, p. 58)

The committee recommended improvements to the quality of the pre-registration year, previously the intern year, which was a responsibility of the GMC. A two-tier registration system was proposed: the first included all those who could be a doctor, and a second tier was to register those who had successfully completed specialist training, including general practice.

A major area of concern was in regard to fitness-to-practice issues and in particular the lack of processes to manage sick doctors. Up to that point, the sick doctor could only be dealt with under serious professional misconduct policies and then labeled as a "bad doctor", as opposed to being ill. The Committee recommended that the GMC introduce new health procedures for these cases.

The Committee agreed with the profession's demands and recommended increased medical representation on the GMC Council, with the number of members increasing to 98.

The Committee did consider the issue of what was called re-certification or re-licensing (revalidation in today's terms) but recommended that there should be no changes in the approach to regulation, and that any re-licensing schemes should only be introduced if there was sound evidence of their effectiveness. So, the status quo remained in that once a doctor had initial registration they would remain on the register as long as the annual license fee was paid. There was no requirement for a doctor to demonstrate that they were engaged in continuing professional development and were up to date with no concerns about their fitness to practice.

The recommendations of the Merrison Committee led to the 1978 Medical Act, which in turn led to the establishment of the revised GMC Council in 1979. This new Council had four main functions:

1 To register doctors
2 The regulation of basic medical education (medical schools) and to coordinate all stages of medical education
3 To manage fitness-to-practice concerns with new health procedures
4 To provide advice on professional standards and ethics.

The new Council had a wider representation from the profession with increased representation from the business world and academia, with the aim of providing a higher level of external scrutiny.

Changing Public Expectations

Around this time in the late 1970s and into the 1980s the expectations of the public began to change dramatically. The second medical revolution continued apace, with developments in technology and data analysis leading to new approaches to diagnosis and treatments (Foss and Rothenberg 1987).

Throughout the 1980s there was a growing movement against the GMC for its apparent inaction in dealing with "problem doctors". Through a series of articles (Smith 1989) numerous criticisms were laid at the GMC. These included the fact the public did not have a voice in Council, that the membership was predominantly doctors, with some arguing that even those doctors were over-represented by the BMA.

At this time there was a growing sense of public concern about the GMC's ability to deal with poor practice. Kennedy (1981), a non-medical member of the GMC Council, voiced concerns about the accountability of the Council, which was to the Privy Council and not to Parliament itself. In addition, he had concerns about inadequate lay representation and the general lack of scrutiny allowed by the public over the Council's activities. He argued that the GMC had a duty to protect the public interest but it had no processes for obtaining feedback from the public.

Criticism of the GMC came from others within the Council membership itself. Jean Robinson, a lay representative on Council, voiced the patients' views on the inadequacy of the Council's policies on poor clinical practice (Robinson 1988). Her concerns also included the lack of transparency and the GMC's reluctance, or refusal, to effectively address the issue of professional competence. The perception of the GMC was of an organization reluctant to innovate and almost wholly reactive to events and complaints.

The UK Political Landscape 1980–1990

In the 1980s to 1990s the political landscape in the UK changed completely. Margaret Thatcher was Prime Minister from 1979 to 1990, leading a Conservative Government. GP fundholding, a form of internal market, was introduced in 1991 as a result of the Conservative's National Health Service and Community Care Act 1990. With this, GPs took over responsibility for the purchase of all hospital services for their patients. This development was not without its critics, but it has been argued that fundholding brought, for some, new investment into primary care and facilitated better data systems, improved clinical management, and multi-professional clinical audit. Despite these patient-focused improvements, some practices were left in deficit and a two-tier system developed. Fundholding was ceased by the new Labour Government in 1997.

In 1990, the Contract was introduced for GPs. This was the first step into performance-managing GPs as independent contractors. The contract, despite being rejected by the profession through a national ballot, was imposed by the then Health Secretary, Kenneth Clarke. Within the new contractual arrangements, GPs were now required to undertake health checks with newly registered patients, those over 75, and patients who had not seen a GP within three years. New fees and allowances were introduced including for child health surveillance and minor surgery services. This performance-based approach, although resisted by the profession, did have the effect of increasing GP involvement in health promotion (Boyce et al. 2010).

Case Drivers for Change

Throughout the early 1990s, there were increasing concerns in the pubic and in the profession generated by a number of high-profile cases of malpractice. There was a sense that self-regulation was at risk and was not likely to be sustainable. The GMC, in a series of booklets under the general heading *Duties of a Doctor*, published a code of good practice, the first version of Good Medical Practice. This publication set out for the first time standards in competence, care and conduct (General Medical Council 1995). When first published this code was "advisory" but was embedded into all aspects of registration in 1998. This led on to a decision in 1999 by the GMC that all doctors who were practicing should have their practice evaluated on a regular basis.

A series of scandals in the NHS involving doctors and the public outcry associated with each, acted as case drivers for change. A number of these will be explored briefly. They include:

1 **The Gosport Review**
2 **Bristol Royal Infirmary**
3 **Alder Hey Children's Hospital**
4 **Clifford Ayling**
5 **Richard Neale**
6 **Harold Shipman**

The Gosport Review

Through 1991 and 1992 concerns were raised on multiple occasions by nursing staff on the elderly care wards at Gosport War Memorial Hospital, Portsmouth. The concerns centered around the opiate prescribing practices of Dr Barton, a Clinical Assistant, and also a GP who managed the wards on a day-to-day basis. These concerns were made in writing with support from a Royal College of Nursing representative to the hospital managers. No action was taken.

Further complaints were made in 1998, which led to an internal investigation by the Trust but again, no action was taken. The family then reported their concerns to the local police but these were not investigated. Several other patient concerns were raised with the hospital and the police in 1999, and this led to the Trust asking for an external review by the Commission for Health Improvement (CHI), in 2001.

The CHI report in 2002 stated:

> a number of factors . . . contributed to a failure of trust systems to ensure good quality patient care:
>
> there were insufficient local prescribing guidelines in place governing the prescription of powerful pain relieving and sedative medicines;
>
> the lack of a rigorous, routine review of pharmacy data [which] led to high levels of prescribing on wards caring for older people not being questioned;
>
> the absence of adequate trust wide supervision and appraisal systems [which] meant that poor prescribing practice was not identified;
>
> there was a lack of thorough multidisciplinary total patient assessment to determine care needs on admission.
>
> (Commission for Health Improvement 2002, p. vii)

Eventually an Independent Panel was commissioned and found that in the 1990s the lives of more than 450 patients were shortened by the prescribing and administering of dangerous doses of medication, particularly opiates, by Dr Barton. The panel also concluded that it was clear that concerns were raised by nursing staff and by families on several occasions, but these concerns were not addressed in any meaningful way.

In 2010 the GMC found Dr Barton guilty of serious professional misconduct and of putting her patients at risk of an early death. However, the GMC took into account her 10 years of safe practice as a GP and did not erase her from the register. Instead, a number of conditions were placed on her practice. Following several police investigations, the Crown Prosecution Service concluded in 2010 that no criminal charges were to be brought after finding insufficient evidence of gross negligence manslaughter. Dr Barton subsequently retired in 2011 and relinquished her GMC registration.

The Government's response to The Right Reverend James Jones' report came in November 2018, entitled *Learning from Gosport* (Department of Health and Social Care 2018). The key recommendations for the Trust were all designed to minimize the chance of something similar happening again.

In the Foreword to the report the Reverend Jones makes damming comment on a number of organizations, including the GMC, who failed to act to protect patients:

> . . .*when relatives complained about the safety of patients and the appropriateness of their care, they were consistently let down by those in authority – both individuals and institutions. These included the senior management of the hospital, healthcare organisations, Hampshire Constabulary, local politicians, the coronial system, the Crown Prosecution Service, the General Medical Council and the Nursing and Midwifery Council. All failed to act in ways that would have better protected patients and relatives, whose interests some subordinated to the reputation of the hospital and the professions involved.*
>
> (Gosport War Memorial Hospital 2018, p. viii)

Bristol Royal Infirmary

When the scandal of high mortality rates at the Bristol Royal Infirmary (BRI) pediatric cardiac surgery unit began to be reported in 1998, there was a wave of anger directed at the GMC. The Report of the Public Inquiry into children's heart surgery at the BRI 1984–1995 was published in 2001 (Department of Health 2001). The Report concluded that between 30 and 35 children undergoing heart surgery at BRI died between 1991 and 1995 who would in all probability have survived if treated elsewhere. The mortality at BRI at the time for children aged one and under was double that compared with England as a whole, and even higher for neonates. Around a third of children who underwent open heart surgery received inadequate care.

The inquiry report described a flawed system of care with poor teamwork between professionals, "too much power in too few hands." A key finding was the surgeons at the center of the scandal lacked any insight into their behavior. Although there were failings of these individual surgeons, there were also inadequacies at every point in the patient pathway from referral to diagnosis, surgical intervention and immediate post-operative care.

When the BRI Inquiry Report was published it marked another major turning point in the regulation of doctors. The almost daily press coverage of events appalled the public. There was shock that things could have on so for long. A key concern was the fact that so many professionals in the system had been aware of events but had not taken any action.

The two surgeons at the center of the scandal and the Chief Executive Officer (CEO) of BRI (a doctor) were found guilty by the GMC of serious professional misconduct. Dr John Roylance, CEO, appealed and the GMC decision was upheld by the Privy Council. Even some of the GMC's most vocal critics commended their role in the aftermath of the Bristol scandal (Klein 1998). On the other hand, the GMC were the subject of public criticism by the then Health Secretary, Frank Dobson, for only banning the second surgeon, Mr Dhasmana, from operating on children for three years and not erasing him from the medical register.

Alder Hey Children's Hospital

The Royal Liverpool Children's Inquiry Report (2001), referred to as the Redfern Report, as it was chaired by Michael Redfern, Queens Council, generated a huge public and political reaction.

The need for this arose from the BRI scandal where it emerged that many organs had been removed and retained for research and teaching. The largest collection was identified at the Royal Liverpool Children's Hospital (Alder Hey Children's Hospital). Organs had been removed and retained without the proper consent of the relatives. The inquiry found that the practice of organ removal and retention was widespread and that the medical profession had an extremely paternalistic approach, believing that the parents would not wish to know about the retention and/or the use to which the organs might be put.

The inquiry uncovered full-scale systematic removal of organs from 1988 to 1995. Every child who had a post-mortem had tissue samples or whole organs removed, but in general these were not used for teaching or research and remained stored. The inquiry came to the conclusion that a significant proportion of the responsibility lay with Dick van Velzen, a Dutch pathologist, who was Chair of Pathology over the relevant years.

Van Velzen left Alder Hey in 1995 to work in IWK Grace Hospital in Nova Scotia, Canada, but was then sacked from his role in 1998.

Following publication of the Redfern Report, van Velzen's UK registration was temporarily suspended by the GMC. In July 2001 he was convicted of improperly storing human body parts of a child whilst working in Halifax and received a 12-month probation order. In December 2004 the Crown Prosecution Service in the UK decided not to prosecute van Velzen and in June 2005 the GMC erased him from the medical register.

The inquiry concluded that despite numerous opportunities, neither the Trust nor the University addressed complaints about Van Velzen, and as a result of systemic inaction he was allowed to continue to act unethically and illegally for years.

This was another example of the "doctor knows best" attitude and further evidence of the medical and health system colluding to cover up and not deal with malpractice.

There were hundreds of press articles around this time, reporting the public's shock and disgust. These feelings were fuelled by reports of the trauma experienced by relatives and parents.

The public, professionals, and politicians all acknowledged wrongdoing at Alder Hey Hospital and agreed that the practices of the past needed to change. The Alder Hey report was a catalyst to that process of change, particularly with regard to the procedures for obtaining consent to post-mortems, and retaining tissue and organ samples for use in education and research. The most significant outcome from this inquiry was the passing of new legislation, the Human Tissue Act 2004, setting out in law the requirements for informed consent and procedures for storing and use of human tissue.

Then on 13 July 2001 the Secretary of State for Health announced the setting up of three separate, independent statutory inquiries, none of which was to be held in public. One of those inquiries related to Clifford Ayling, the second to Richard Neale, a Consultant Obstetrician and Gynecologist who worked in a number of hospitals in North Yorkshire, and the third to William Kerr and Michael Haslam, two Consultant Psychiatrists who practiced in North Yorkshire. We shall briefly explore the former two inquiries. These inquiries had broadly similar terms of reference, which required in each case an investigation of how the local NHS and other organizations had handled complaints about the performance and/or conduct of the doctors.

Clifford Ayling

In 1998 Clifford Ayling, working as a GP, was arrested on charges of indecent assault on former patients. In December 2000 he was found guilty of 12 counts of indecent assault relating to ten female patients and received a four-year custodial sentence. His name was placed indefinitely on the sex offender's register under the Sex Offenders Act 1997. He was acquitted of a further nine charges and 14 others were ordered to lie on the file.

On 15 June 2001 the professional conduct committee of the GMC determined that Ayling's name should be erased from the medical register. In 2002, Dame Anna Pauffley was appointed to chair an Independent Investigation into how the NHS handled allegations about Ayling's conduct (Department of Health 2004).

Clifford Ayling qualified in 1963 and worked in hospitals around London, including the North Middlesex Hospital, from 1971 to 1973. From 1974 until 1988 he was employed as a part-time clinical assistant in obstetrics and gynecology, working at the Kent and Canterbury Hospital in Canterbury and the Isle of Thanet Hospital in Margate.

In 1981 he entered general practice in Folkestone, and from 1984 until 1994, he was also employed as a part-time clinical assistant in colposcopy at the William Harvey Hospital in Ashford. He also undertook locum medical sessions in family planning clinics in east Kent.

The complaints that led to Ayling's convictions for sexual assault related to inappropriate touching or examinations of women's breasts or gynecological examination. The earliest incident considered in the criminal trial took place in 1991, and most incidents occurred in the GP's surgery, rather than in hospitals. It was a central part of Ayling's defense in the criminal trial that the disputed examinations were medically necessary. This argument was dismissed by the jury, and Ayling was found guilty on all 12 counts.

There was extensive press coverage at the time. The *Guardian* newspaper, in an article online on 29 April 2002, reported details of the traumatic experiences of some of the women, quoting one victim as saying:

> *all down the line, women weren't listened to.*

> (Bosley 2002)

The *Daily Mail* reported on a landmark court case where Ayling was ordered to pay over £250 000 in compensation to his victims (Rayner 2002). The article reported some of the horrific details that the victims had to endure and the long-term psychological damage caused.

Richard Neale

The case of the gynecologist Richard Neale added further to the public's concern about the GMC. The inquiry found serious acts of omission of behalf of the GMC and served to highlight their ineffective reactive approach to poorly performing doctors. Neale qualified in London in 1970, and following a house officer job at Westminster Hospital, obtained full GMC registration in 1971. He then worked briefly as a GP in Cheshire from 1972 to 1974. He moved to Canada in 1977, working firstly in British Columbia and then in Ontario. In 1978 he performed a high-risk operation on a patient who subsequently died, and as a result, in 1979, he lost his hospital privileges. He was required to undergo further training or cease practice. In 1981 he was working at Oshawa Hospital in Ontario, Canada, when a patient died following treatment by Neale. In 1985 he was erased from the Canadian Medical Register following a disciplinary hearing into the death of this patient.

However, in 1984, Neale commenced employment in the Yorkshire Regional Health Authority working at the Friarage Hospital and Darlington Memorial Hospital. In 1992, following reorganization of the NHS, his employment was transferred to the Northallerton Health Services NHS Trust, and that year he was appointed Clinical Director of Obstetrics and Gynecology. In 1993, media stories emerged revealing that Neale had been struck off in Canada in 1985 and had made a failed application for reinstatement there in 1987. In December 1993 the Trust investigated these allegations. In January 1994, as a result of not disclosing the fact he had been struck off in Canada, he was removed from the post of Clinical Director, but was allowed to continue clinical practice. In 1995 the Trust made the decision to set up a disciplinary hearing into various allegations concerning Neale's conduct and clinical competence. Neale contested all the allegations and a decision was made to offer him a severance package. After a year's sabbatical, Neale left the Trust's employment on 30 November 1996. He was then employed at the Leicester Royal Infirmary NHS Trust between November 1995 and March 1996, and St Mary's Hospital, Isle of Wight for two periods between April and July 1996.

On 25 July 2000, the General Medical Council erased Neale's name from the register after being found guilty of professional misconduct.

The press coverage of the Neale case reported that the North Yorkshire Police had written to the GMC about Neale in 1988 but no action was taken. The Independent Investigation (Department of Health 2004) found that the GMC were fully aware of his erasure in Canada and also of a police caution accepted by Neale in 1993 following an incident at a public toilet. The GMC were directly accused of having failed in their responsibility to act.

All of these cases were prominent in the press over a relatively short space of time. There were the recurrent themes of criminal activity, clinical incompetence, the individuals concerned not having insight, the system being aware of allegations, typically over a long period of time, and no action been taken. Criticism was again laid at the GMC for not having systems to assess clinical competence, allowing individual doctors to harm patients.

These cases and others had a major impact on the public's perception of the closed paternalistic system that doctors were operating in. Then another single case, that of Harold Shipman, came to light and acted as the single most important catalyst for change.

Harold Shipman

Harold Shipman was a single-handed GP working in Donneybrook Medical Centre in Hyde, Manchester. The scandal of Shipman first began to surface in 1998 when concerns were raised by Dr Linda Reynolds, a local GP in Hyde, about the high death rate of Shipman's patients. She also had concerns about the high numbers of cremation forms for elderly women that Shipman needed countersigned. The police became involved but decided there was insufficient evidence to investigate further.

Shipman's last victim was Mrs Kathleen Grundy, who was found dead at her home in June 1998. He was the last person to see her alive and signed her death certificate stating old age as the cause of death. Mrs Gundy's daughter, Angela Woodruff, became concerned when she was informed that her mother had made out a new will leaving her estate, valued at £360 000, to Shipman. Angela Woodruff went to the police, who began an investigation and her mother's body was exhumed and was found to contain traces of morphine.

The police investigated other deaths Shipman had certified. They discovered a pattern of his administering lethal doses of diamorphine, signing patients' death certificates, and then falsifying medical records to indicate that they had been in poor health. Shipman was arrested in September 1998, and subsequently found guilty of the murder of 15 patients. In all probability he was responsible for the murder of over 200 individuals.

Dame Janet Smith chaired the Shipman Inquiry and in her fifth report (The Shipman Inquiry 2004) she considered the GMC proposals set out in the previous consultation for the introduction of revalidation. So although the response had been generally positive to the proposals, following Dame Janet's report there were some who reflected that the proposals put forward by the GMC in 2000 were completely inadequate. Roger Neighbour, the then President of the RCGP, stated:

> *The GMC's proposals pre-Dame Janet, much as we might wish them to have been adequate, were more appropriate to a golf club's membership committee than to a profession.*
>
> (Neighbour 2005, p. 241)

The next step on the journey to the current revalidation process was in June 2000, when the GMC published a consultation document on their proposals for the revalidation process (GMC 2000). The GMC received many responses to this consultation, most of which were broadly supportive of the principles of revalidation. Almost all respondents approved the idea of a link between appraisal and revalidation. There were, however, concerns about the high level of support doctors would require to ensure the process was meaningful. There was a consistent view of the importance of ensuring that the developmental nature of appraisal was not lost. There was also concern about the total cost to roll out and provide ongoing administrative support for the revalidation process. Assurances were sought that this cost would not fall to individual doctors. It was suggested that the proposals should be tested in pilot sites and any evaluation should include a cost–benefit analysis.

In 2001 the GMC introduced the requirement for annual appraisal for doctors, and in 2002 the Medical Act 1983 (amendment order 2002), introduced the concept of revalidation into the legislation for the first time.

Good Doctors: Safer Patients

As a result of the Shipman Inquiries, the work on medical revalidation was paused and the then Chief Medical Officer for England, Sir Liam Donaldson, was asked to undertake a major review of medical regulation (Department of Health 2006). In this, he discussed the background to regulation and made proposals for change in the regulatory framework in order to assure and improve the performance of doctors to protect the public.

This review was commissioned by the Secretary of State for Health following the fifth Shipman report where Dame Janet Smith specifically criticized the GMC's proposal to rely on annual appraisals of doctors and questioned whether this process would in reality be a rigorous assessment of a doctor's fitness to practice. So at that point, the question remained as to whether annual appraisal cycles were an effective mechanism to identify doctors who were delivering a poor quality of care or were incompetent.

In his report Donaldson considered a number of high-risk industries and explored the regulatory processes in place at that time for civil aviation pilots who undertook competency checks every six months and an annual renewal of their license. He also considered nuclear power unit desk engineers and air traffic controllers. He described a number of common themes in these three high-risk industries as below:

1 Independent regulators
2 Regular formal proficiency checks – using direct observation and simulation
3 Assessments made against clearly defined standards of competence
4 A focus on non-technical skills being assessed – situational awareness, leadership, communication and team working
5 A remedial and retraining approach to "failure"
6 Regular health checks and random drug and alcohol screening.

Although acknowledging that these processes were rigorous, Donaldson argued that the transferability of these into medicine was not practical. He argued that as a result of the scale of the number of doctors (at that time 170 000) compared with 17 000 pilots, the logistics of using a similar process in medicine would not be feasible.

Donaldson also argued that the cost of replicating a similar process that pilots were subject to would be prohibitive and unjustifiable. There would also need to be evidence that any new revised process is safer for patients.

Donaldson also stated that in these other high-risk industries, failure to perform can have a direct impact of the individual's safety and that of co-workers as well as the public. In medicine, however, the consequences of failure in performance of the doctor fall on a third party, the patient.

The counter-argument is that doctors are still in such a privileged and trusted position and in general, even today with clinical governance processes, national morbidity audits and other processes, it is still not inconceivable that another Shipman event could happen.

Donaldson made a total of 44 recommendations and the key actions included:

> *major changes to the structure, functions and governance of the General Medical Council;*
>
> *extension of the processes of medical regulation to the local level to create a stronger interface with the health care system;*
>
> *the creation of a clear, unambiguous and operationalized standard to define a good doctor, and its adoption into the contracts of all doctors;*
>
> *measures to reduce the risk of poorly performing doctors falling through the net, especially since the expansion in the diversity of roles, working patterns and practice settings;*
>
> *steps to further the consistency with which medical education is managed across undergraduate and postgraduate curricula;*
>
> *processes to bring medical students within the scope of medical regulation and to further assure the quality of all doctors upon initial employment, irrespective of their place of qualification;*
>
> *improve access for the public to timely and meaningful information about doctors, coupled with measures to ensure that such information is handled intelligently.*

(Department of Health 2006, p. xiv)

The response from the profession to Donaldson's report was generally positive, and it was described as "ground breaking" (Pringle 2006). Donald Irvine, former President of the GMC from 1995 to 2002, commended the report and called for the GMC Council to be disbanded so that a refreshed membership could take things forward (Irvine 2006).

The next step in the journey was the publication of a White Paper in 2007 (Department of Health 2007). As a result of changes in public and professional opinion, the White Paper concluded that it was no longer acceptable to assume that any health professional continued to be fit to practice without evidence. It was again argued that what was required was a level of assurance for the public. In the White Paper, the Government proposed that there would be two main components for all health care professionals to revalidate. The first was relicensing, which required all professionals to demonstrate that they remained fit to practice, and a second process of recertification that would only apply to specialist doctors and GPs. These groups would need to demonstrate that they remained competent in their specialty.

Following the White Paper, the report of the Chief Medical Officer for England's Working Group was published in July 2008 and set out the key principles for implementing medical revalidation (Department of Health 2008a). These had been agreed between the Department of Health, the Academy of Medical Royal Colleges and the GMC. These proposals described two processes. The first was that all licensed doctors had to confirm that they were practicing in accordance with the GMC's generic standards (relicensing). The second was in reference to those doctors practicing as GPs or who were on the Specialist Register who would have to confirm they meet the standards appropriate for their specialty (recertification).

The Darzi Report

Another landmark on this journey was the publication of Lord Darzi's report, *High Quality Care for All* (Department of Health 2008b). The review involved thousands of clinical, social care and health service professionals and members of the public. The purpose of the report was to focus on what the NHS could do to improve the prevention of ill health in partnership with other authorities and agencies. At the heart of the report was an emphasis on quality, which was defined as safe, effective and efficient care. The focus should be on personalized care led by local changes.

Darzi proposed a stronger role for the National Institute for Health and Clinical Excellence (NICE). The review suggested that all patients would receive treatments approved by NICE if recommended by clinicians. Darzi articulated the importance of focusing on outcomes rather than targets. The proposal was that targets such as 18-week waits that were once considered aspirational would become established as minimum standards. In the future, national challenges would be met through minimum standards and commissioning (in England only).

Darzi also recommended the need for a renewed focus on primary care, with proposals to establish multi-professional polyclinics and a focus on the importance of patient choice and preference.

With regard to regulation, the review highlighted the role of the new joint regulator in England – the Care Quality Commission (CQC). The report noted that the CQC would have increased enforcement powers compared with its predecessor regulators, suggesting that the CQC would have a stronger focus on compliance and more flexible powers to deal with those providers not meeting registration requirements.

Darzi was broadly supportive of professional revalidation, but commented that for any change to be effective it would need to meet patients' needs and be driven by clinicians themselves.

The UK Revalidation Programme Board

The UK Revalidation Programme Board (UKRPB) was established in 2009 chaired by Sir Keith Pearson. The purpose of the UKRPB was to provide advice to the GMC during the implementation phase of revalidation in order to support the GMC in meeting its regulatory objectives. The Board had high-level oversight and leadership of the development of revalidation across the four nations in the UK, to ensure as much as possible that there was a consistent approach. The core membership comprised representatives from across the four UK health departments, Royal Colleges, the BMA and individuals providing the patients' voice.

In March 2010 the GMC proposed further changes suggesting that revalidation should be one single system as opposed to what had been proposed previously, a two-stage process for relicensing and recertification. The rationale for a single system was that it would be more effective and efficient. This consultation was extensive, involving doctors, employers and patient groups, and the response was published in October that year (General Medical Council 2010) with the key proposals as:

- Revalidation would be based on a single set of processes for assessing doctors' fitness to practice
- This evaluation should be based on a continuing assessment of doctors' performance in the workplace
- There would be a network of Responsible Officers – all of them senior licensed doctors – who will make recommendations on whether or not doctors will be revalidated
- The Medical Royal Colleges and Faculties would not be directly involved in making recommendations – a major change from previous proposals
- All doctors in training would revalidate through their engagement with training requirements
- The Medical Register would state the field of practice on the basis of which a doctor has secured revalidation.

In order to understand the benefits and logistics, and to gather the views of doctors, a series of ten Pathfinder Pilots were established between March and April 2011. These were subject to an independent evaluation by Frontline Consultants and Durham University. Over 3000 doctors in primary and secondary care took part in strengthened appraisals. The key findings were:

- Ninety-six percent of pilot organizations stated that they expected revalidation to lead to improved patient care, with 82% of them expecting improved patient safety
- Eighty percent of organizations also expected improvement in the patient experience.

When the GMC's consultation was launched, it was intended that revalidation would be "live" in 2011, but under political pressure the GMC decided to defer the launch until late in 2012 to enable further information to be gathered from the pilot sites so that there would be a better understanding of the costs, benefits and practicalities of implementation.

The Responsible Officer Regulations

In 2010 the Responsible Officer (RO) regulations were enacted across the UK. These set out the roles and responsibilities for ROs and their designated bodies. Please see Chapter 4 for more detail on the practical implications of these.

Revalidation is Launched

On the 3 December 2012, revalidation formally began, and when launched the GMC Chairman, Peter Rubin, said:

> This is the biggest change in medical regulation since 1858. We are leading the world.
>
> (White 2012)

Set against this major development in medical regulation, high-profile cases of poor care and malpractice at a systems and individual practitioner level continued to hit the press.

The Report of the Mid Staffordshire NHS Foundation Trust Public Inquiry (Francis 2013) identified systems failures across the Trust and the wider clinical, education and training governance arrangements. These failures led to increased mortality and appalling care in Stafford Hospital between 2005 and 2008. The report made a total of 290 recommendations. With regard to fitness-to-practice issues, recommendation number 222 stated:

> The General Medical Council should have a clear policy about the circumstances in which a generic complaint or report ought to be made to it, enabling a more proactive approach to monitoring fitness to practice.
>
> (Francis 2013, p. 108)

The Francis report put further pressure on the GMC to reconsider fitness-to-practice processes and to be more proactive in managing these, and contributed to the shifting context in which medical revalidation was being developed and rolled out across the UK.

The King's Fund 2013

In 2013 The King's Fund was commissioned by the NHS Revalidation Support team to undertake a qualitative assessment of the impact of revalidation on the behavior of doctors and the impact on the culture of NHS organizations (Nath et al. 2014). Although the study was based on seven sites in England, it could be argued that the findings applied equally across the UK. The sites participating were two primary care areas, two secondary care trusts, a mental health trust, an independent provider, and a locum agency. The total sample was almost 5500 doctors.

A small sample of appraisers, appraisees, ROs, a CEO, a non-executive director, a HR director, a Nurse Director and a patient representative were included. The methodology used focus groups and one-to-one interviews. In total, the research team spoke to 126 individuals, with 90 doctors and appraisers, and 36 patient representatives.

The recommendations were:

1　Strengthen and refine the existing process
Retain those elements that are working well, including doctors' engagement with annual appraisal, reflection on their scope of practice and contribution to quality improvement.

2　Unlock the potential for Quality Improvement
Additional guidance and support is needed to allow individuals to engage with clinical governance and quality improvement embedded into their appraisals. To enable this to continue and move forward, organizations need to provide the resources. A key element is moving to a position where the benefits of revalidation are seen and understood at the organizational and national level.

At an individual level all doctors must keep an open mind to the potential for the revalidation process to lead to improvement in the care they provide to patients.

3　Embed a culture of learning
At a systems level, leaders should encourage doctors to benchmark themselves against comparators. To achieve this, accurate data is needed, with enablers and encouragement for all doctors to engage with audit and develop systems whereby best practice can be shared across organizations. Patient and peer feedback is essential and there is a need to ensure mechanisms are in place to act this on. This applies equally at organizational level. The authors summarized:

> Our view is that medical revalidation, with the right conditions, can be a valuable driver of behaviour and cultures that support sustained quality improvement. The time to develop those conditions is now.

Above all, leaders should bear in mind that large scale change requires them to have the tenacity and vision to create a process that is valued by all who are involved in it. As we have previously stated, what is of most value is what is practised when no-one is watching.

(Nath et al. 2014, p. 27)

The Pearson Review

In 2016 Sir Keith Pearson was asked by the GMC to undertake a review of revalidation (Pearson 2017). At that point, revalidation had been live for four years and the majority of doctors in the UK had undergone one cycle, so it was felt an opportune time to review the process.

The terms of reference were very broad and were designed to enable an assessment of the available evidence on the operation and impact of revalidation. A wide range of data sources was used, including data held by the GMC, any published work on the impact, and feedback from a range of organizations such as Royal Colleges, the BMA, NHS England and patient groups.

Pearson's summary of the current position included:

- Revalidation has ensured that the appraisal process covers the whole scope of practice of doctors
- Reflection on a range of feedback, including patient feedback, is starting to change doctors' practice
- Revalidation has strengthened clinical governance helping heath care organizations to identify poorly performing doctors and provide help and support for them
- The principles of revalidation are sound, but more local support for doctors is needed to ensure the process is less burdensome.

Pearson expressed concern about those doctors who are practicing outside of a managed environment or those who change jobs and location frequently. He highlighted the need for more work to be done to ensure increased public awareness of revalidation. He also flagged the need for action to be taken to make it easier for patients to provide feedback to doctors.

He considered that revalidation did not need a major overhaul and that in general it was working well, and his recommendations were aimed at improving certain elements of the process.

The GMC accepted all of Pearson's recommendations and in July 2017 set out their *Taking Revalidation Forward Action Plan* (GMC 2017). This plan was organized into six work streams each covering a priority area from the Pearson report:

- Making revalidation more accessible to patients and the public
- Reducing burdens and improving the appraisal experience for doctors

- Strengthening assurance where doctors work in multiple locations
- Reducing the number of doctors without a connection
- Tracking the impact of revalidation
- Supporting improved governance.

UK Medical Revalidation Evaluation coLLAboration (UMbRELLA) Study

One of the action points under tracking the impact of revalidation was to review the conclusion of the UMbRELLA study. In 2014 the GMC commissioned a consortium, the UK Medical Revalidation Evaluation coLLAboration (UMbRELLA), to explore the regulatory impacts of revalidation (UMbRELLA 2018). Between 2014 and 2017, the consortium used a mixed-methods approach to assess the impact and consequences, both intended and unintended, of the implementation of revalidation over this timescale to help inform future developments. This was a comprehensive study involving a range of approaches including undertaking nine literature reviews, surveying over 85 000 doctors, recording 44 appraisals and interviews of 156 doctors and patient representatives.

The key findings were:

- The process of revalidation based on cycles of annual appraisal has been widely implemented but the impact of revalidation is uncertain
- There is a need to provide further guidance to a group of doctors who have significant non-clinical roles, as confusion still exists about what the full scope of practice entails
- There are higher deferral rates in black ethnic minority groups compared to white and this differential attainment needs further research.

The study reported that there remains uncertainty in medical and patient organizations as to the aim of revalidation. The authors reflected that there is a danger that the process for doctors is seen as a series of tasks in order to be able to complete the documentation. This tick-box type of approach may be being facilitated by some of the IT systems supporting appraisal.

The authors were clear in stating that central to the impact of appraisal, particularly about positive change in doctors' behavior, was the role of the appraiser. On the basis of this, they recommended resource allocation should focus on further up-skilling appraisers in mentoring and coaching techniques. This study also confirmed the ongoing challenges in patients being able to provide meaningful feedback to support the appraisal process.

Chapter Summary

In this chapter we have explored the recent history of the evolution of regulation of doctors in the UK. This evolution has been driven by many factors. The expectations of the general public have increased immeasurably from the 1990s. This has been driven by the third medical revolution, underpinned by the internet allowing ease of access to information, and the smart phone. A series of high-profile cases, including Shipman, have acted as case drivers exposing the weaknesses in the old system whereby there were no processes to assure a doctor's ongoing fitness to practice or his/her competence to undertake what was expected of them in their day-to-day practice. Over this period of time the system has moved from a doctor simply paying the GMC an annual retention fee as the sole process for maintaining one's licence/registration to a position of annual appraisal, and on a five-year cycle a RO making a recommendation to the GMC. The movement to the current process has been tortuous, with many twists along the journey.

The social contract with the public has changed, and the rise of patient-reported experience and outcome measures as being pivotal to service redesign is to be welcomed. These and other changes, it was hoped, should encourage a move away from the "doctor knows best" and paternalistic approach of the profession exemplified by the BRI and Alder Hey Children's Hospital scandals.

There are changing expectations of patients, government, NHS managers, and regulators. The traditional image and perception of the medical profession has changed from that in the past. It has always been the case, but today there is even more focus on doctors and all health care workers putting the wellbeing of patients as their prime responsibility. There is an expectation that doctors are technically competent, open and honest. The challenge is that there is a perception that these qualities have been eroded or diluted from or in the profession. As a result, doctors now have to earn the respect of patients, which in turn affords them their professional status and the societal privileges that come with that.

The general population have transformed in their expectations. A public survey of nearly 2000 people in 2017 reported that 44% thought that the standard of care in the NHS had got worse in the previous year (Ipsos MORI 2017).

The public expect the service to be convenient and easy for them to access and to be responsive to their needs. In addition, patients increasingly expect to participate in the decision-making process. The model of service delivery has changed. There is increasing organizational control over doctors' work, the workload, and hence the way doctors now practice. There are continuous cycles of ongoing government reform. In the UK since 1999 all health matters have been devolved. As a result, there are different and constantly diverging health care systems at play across Northern Ireland, Scotland, Wales and England.

There has also been a sea-change in the way doctors are expected to interact with other professionals. This includes the emergence of the Multi-Disciplinary Team (MDT) as being responsible for coordinating and planning the provision of care for many patients in a wide range of care pathways. In addition, there has been a wide diversification of roles, with the perception of the erosion of the doctor's traditional role as the lead of the clinical team with new roles such as the Physician Associate.

As a result, the social contract that the medical profession has with society is changing more than at any point in the past. The social contract (compact) is being renegotiated with the patient at the center of practice. This in turn requires strong and skillful medical leadership with a redefining of doctors' roles.

References

Bosley, S. (2002). How did he get away with it for so long? *The Guardian*. https://www.theguardian.com/society/2002/apr/29/medicineandhealth.lifeandhealth (accessed 7 May 2021).

Boyce, T., Peckham, S. Hann, A. et al. (2010). *A pro-active approach. Health Promotion and Ill-health Prevention*. London: The King's Fund. https://www.kingsfund.org.uk/sites/default/files/field/field_document/health-promotion-ill-health-prevention-gp-inquiry-research-paper-mar11.pdf (accessed 7 May 2021).

British Medical Association (1965). *A Charter for the Family Doctor Service*. London: BMA.

Collings, J.S. (1950). General practice in England today: a reconnaissance. *Lancet* **1**: 555–585.

Commission for Health Improvement (2002). *Investigation into the Portsmouth Healthcare NHS Trust. Gosport War Memorial Hospital*. Norwich: The Stationery Office. https://www.gosportpanel.independent.gov.uk/document-library/documents/SOH004374/ (accessed 7 May 2021).

Department of Health (2001). The report of the public inquiry into children's heart surgery at the Bristol Royal Infirmary 1984–1995: learning from Bristol. Cm 5207(ii). London: Department of Health. https://webarchive.nationalarchives.gov.uk/20100407202126/http://www.dh.gov.uk/en/Publicationsandstatistics/Publications/PublicationsPolicyAndGuidance/DH_4009387 (accessed 7 May 2021).

Department of Health (2004). *Committee of Inquiry to Investigate How the NHS Handled Allegations About the Performance and Conduct of Richard Neale*. Cm 6315. London: The Stationery Office.

Department of Health (2006). Good doctors, safer patients. Proposals to strengthen the system to assure and improve the performance of doctors and to protect the safety of patients. A report by the Chief Medical Officer. London: Department of Health. https://webarchive.nationalarchives.gov.uk/20080728114331/http://www.dh.gov.uk/en/Publicationsandstatistics/Publications/PublicationsPolicyAndGuidance/DH_4137232 (accessed 7 May 2021).

Department of Health (2007). *Trust, Assurance and Safety: The Regulation of Health Care Professionals in the 21st century*. Cm 7013. London: The Stationery Office.

Department of Health (2008b). *High Quality Care for All: NHS Next Stage Review Final Report*. Cm 7432. London: The Stationery Office. https://www.gov.uk/government/publications/high-quality-care-for-all-nhs-next-stage-review-final-report (accessed 7 May 2021).

Foss, L. and Rothenberg, K. (1987). The second Medical revolution. *Theoretical Medicine* **18**: 319–322.

General Medical Council (1995). *Duties of a Doctor*. London: GMC.

General Medical Council (2000). *Revalidating Doctors: Ensuring Standards, Securing the Future*. London: GMC.

General Medical Council (2010). *Revalidation: The Way Ahead. Response to Our Consultation*. London: GMC.

General Medical Council (2017). *Taking Revalidation Forward Action Plan*. https://www.gmc-uk.org/-/media/documents/rt---taking-revalidation-forward-action-plan---dc10267_pdf-71185817.pdf (accessed 7 May 2021).

General Medical Council (2019). *The State of Medical Education and Practice in the UK*. London: GMC.

Gosport War Memorial Hospital (2018). *The Report of the Gosport Independent Panel*. House of Commons. HC 1084. https://www.gosportpanel.independent.gov.uk/media/documents/070618_CCS207_CCS03183220761_Gosport_Inquiry_Whole_Document.pdf (accessed 7 May 2021).

Ipsos MORI (2017). Polling for The Health Foundation. https://www.ipsos.com/ipsos-mori/en-uk/polling-health-foundation-0 (accessed 25 May 2021).

Irvine, D. (2003). *The Doctors' Tale. Professionalism and Public Trust*. Boca Raton, FL: CRC Press.

Irvine, D. (2006). Good doctors: safer patients – the Chief Medical Officer's prescription for regulating doctors. *Journal of the Royal Society of Medicine* **99** (9): 430–432. https://doi.org/10.1177/014107680609900902.

Kennedy, I. (1981). *The Unmasking of Medicine*. London: Allen and Unwin.

Klein, R. (1998). *Regulating the Medical Profession; Doctors and the Public Interest. Health Care UK 1997/98*. London: The King's Fund.

Nath, V., Seale, B., and Kaur, M. (2014). *Medical Revalidation. From Compliance to Commitment*. London: The King's Fund.

Neighbour, R. (2005). Rotten apples. *British Journal of General Practice* **55**: 241.

Pearson, K. (2017). *Taking revalidation forward. Improving the process of relicensing for doctors*. Manchester: General Medical Council. https://www.gmc-uk.org/-/media/documents/Taking_revalidation_forward___Improving_the_process_of_relicensing_for_doctors.pdf_68683704.pdf (accessed 5 May 2021).

Pringle, M. (2006). Regulation and revalidation of doctors. England's chief Medical Officer's report should resolve the uncertainty. *British Medical Journal* **333**: 161–162.

Robinson, J. (1988). *A Patient Voice at the GMC: A Lay Member's View of the General Medical Council*. London: Health Rights.

Royal Liverpool Children's Inquiry (2001). *Report/The Royal Liverpool Children's Inquiry*. London: The Stationery Office.

Society of Health (1980). The start of the NHS 1948. https://www.sochealth.co.uk/national-health-service/the-sma-and-the-foundation-of-the-national-health-service-dr-leslie-hilliard-1980/the-start-of-the-nhs-1948/ (accessed 8 May 2021).

Rayner, G. (2002). Victims of shamed GP in £256,000 test case victory. *The Daily Mail*. https://www.dailymail.co.uk/health/article-109357/Victims-shamed-GP-256-000-test-case-victory.html (accessed 8 May 2021).

Secretary of State for Social Services (1975). *Report of the Committee of Inquiry into the Regulation of the Medical Profession*. Chairman Dr A.W. Merrison. Cmnd 6018. London: HMSO.

Smith, R. (1989). The day of judgement comes closer. *British Medical Journal* **298**: 1241–1244.

The Shipman Inquiry (2004). *Fifth Report. Safeguarding Patients: Lessons from the Past – Proposals for the Future*. Cm 6394. London: The Stationery Office.

UK Medical Revalidation coLLAboration (2018). *Evaluating the regulatory impact of medical revalidation*. https://www.gmc-uk.org/-/media/documents/umbrella-report-final_pdf-74454378.pdf (accessed 8 May 2021).

White, C. (2012). GMC recommends that revalidation go ahead this year. *British Medical Journal* **345**: e6606. https://doi.org/10.1136/bmj.e6606.

Department of Health (2008a). *Medical Revalidation – Principles and Next Steps. The report of the Chief Medical Officer of England's working group*. https://www.plymouth.ac.uk/uploads/production/document/path/1/1919/CMO_Report_of_Revalidation_2008.pdf (accessed 16 May 2021).

Department of Health and Social Care (2018). *Learning from Gosport. The Government response to the report of the Gosport Independent Panel*. https://assets.publishing.service.gov.uk/government/uploads/system/uploads/attachment_data/file/758062/government-response-to-gosport-independent-panel-report.pdf (accessed 7 May 2021).

Francis, R. (2013). *Report of the Mid Staffordshire NHS Foundation Trust Public Inquiry*. House of Commons. London: The Stationery Office. https://www.gov.uk/government/publications/report-of-the-mid-staffordshire-nhs-foundation-trust-public-inquiry (accessed 7 May 2021).

Chapter 4 Revalidation – The Role of the Appraiser, Responsible Officer and Designated Bodies

Introduction

As discussed in the previous chapter, revalidation for all doctors in the UK was established in December 2012. The current regulations stipulate that all doctors have to provide evidence of fitness to practice by engaging in a process of annual appraisal and similar processes in order for them to continue to have a license to practice.

For those who are working as General Practitioners (GPs), Consultants, Staff and Associate Specialists (SAS), Speciality Doctor grade doctors and Locally Employed Doctors, there is an annual appraisal process which is seen as developmental and the basis of which is reflection in, and on practice. After five annual cycles the designated body (DB) that the individual doctor is linked to through their Responsible Officer (RO) will make a recommendation to the General Medical Council (GMC) for revalidation.

For those holding National Training Numbers there is an agreed UK process whereby the expectation is that these doctors in training will engage fully in their training program, and pivotal to the recommendation for revalidation is the self-declaration Form R in the Annual Review of Competency Progression (ARCP) process.

The central concept of revalidation is that the individual doctor is revalidated against the entire scope and breadth of their practice. As a significant number of doctors are involved in leadership, management and research activity at some level, there is clearly a need for each doctor to understand how they can provide the appropriate supporting information across all aspects of the scope of practice.

How to Succeed at Revalidation, First Edition. Peter Donnelly and Katie Webb.
© 2022 John Wiley & Sons Ltd. Published 2022 by John Wiley & Sons Ltd.

The Good Medical Practice

The GMC published a framework which sets out in broad terms the areas that should be covered in appraisal (GMC 2020). The regulator is clear that all doctors must be familiar with the requirements within Good Medical Practice (GMP) and the explanatory guide that supports it. Within this document the regulator uses two separate terms, the first of which is "you must" and the second is "you should."

"You must" is used for an overriding duty or principle, whereas "you should" is used for when the regulator is providing an explanation of how you will meet the overriding duty. In addition, the "you should" term is also used in relation to a duty or principle that may not apply to all situations or all circumstances. GMP clearly states that for a doctor to maintain their license to practice, they must demonstrate through the revalidation process that they are working across the breadth of their practice in line with the principles and values set out within the guidance. It is clearly stated that serious or persistent failure to follow this guidance will put registration at risk.

The GMC Domains

The GMC domains as stated in GMP are (GMC 2020):
Domain 1. Skills, knowledge and performance
> Develop and maintain your professional performance
> Apply knowledge and experience to practice
> Record your work clearly, accurately and legibly

Domain 2. Safety and quality
> Contribute to and comply with systems to protect patients
> Respond to risks to safety
> Risks posed by your health

Domain 3. Communication, partnership and teamwork
> Communicate effectively
> Work collaboratively with colleagues
> Teaching, training, supporting and assessing
> Continuity and coordination of care
> Establish and maintain partnerships with patients

Domain 4. Maintaining trust
> Show respect for patients
> Treat patients and colleagues fairly and without discrimination
> Act with honesty and integrity

A lot of events and/or interactions will map to a number of domains, and most experiences are complex. There are six types of supporting information (SI) that must be collected by the appraisee (GMC 2020). They are:

- Continuing professional development
- Quality improvement activity
- Significant events or serious incidents
- Feedback from patients
- Feedback from colleagues
- Compliments and complaints

The GMP applies to all doctors including those in formal training programs. In addition, in order to clarify the situation for doctors in training, the GMC produced the Generic Professional Capabilities Framework (GMC 2017). Within this, there are further domains which overlap with GMP that explicitly set out a number of descriptors in each of those domains, in order to help doctors in training and their trainers understand their responsibilities.

For doctors in training in busy training programs, balancing service delivery with learning and training, it can be a challenge to understand how to populate their e-portfolio and provide the level of detail required.

The importance of being a reflective practitioner has been highlighted in a joint statement from all the Chief Executives of the UK statutory regulators of health and social care (Nursing and Midwifery Council 2019). An important extract states:

> *Reflection is the thought process where individuals consider their experiences to gain insights about their whole practice. Reflection supports individuals to continually improve the way they work or the quality of care they give to people. It is a familiar, continuous and routine part of the work of health and care professionals.*
>
> *Opportunities for multi-professional teams to reflect and discuss openly and honestly what has happened when things go wrong should be encouraged. These valuable reflective experiences help to build resilience, improve wellbeing and deepen professional commitment.*

This chapter will describe the processes, roles and responsibilities for the appraiser, the RO and the DB. We will also briefly touch upon the requirements for doctors in training in the UK. Chapter 5 describes the tasks for the appraisee. Recognizing that different systems and approaches are applied across the UK, we will have a generic approach to the description of the process.

This chapter will describe the processes in general terms and also explores the specifics of each of the key players in the revalidation cycle. The cornerstone of revalidation is annual appraisal over a five-year cycle.

The key players are:

1 **The Appraiser**
2 **The Responsible Officer**
3 **The Designated Body**

The Appraiser

The role of the appraiser is to facilitate a successful appraisal for the apprai-see. This is a complex role and it is important to be engaged with ongoing learning and support for this. This point was highlighted in a review of the impact of revalidation commissioned by the GMC (UK Medical Revalidation coLLAboration 2018). There are a wide range of skills and personal attributes that are required, and the reality is that not all doctors, no matter how good they are as clinicians, will necessarily be good appraisers.

The activities, roles and responsibilities of the appraiser can be divided across the process.

  i **Preparation before the meeting**
 ii **Activities in the meeting**
iii **Action post-meeting**

Preparation Before the Appraisal Meeting

The key to any successful high-stakes interaction is preparation. This is vitally important for an appraisal meeting. By their very nature, doctors' roles can be complex and the environments in which they function are highly complex adaptive systems (Pype et al. 2018). The first step as an appraiser is to spend time critically reviewing the information in the doctor's submission. There is no right or wrong sequence to this process as long as the following are covered.

1 Review the doctor's personal and professional details. It is useful to cross-reference with the previous appraisal, if available, to check if these have changed.

2 Within the professional details a key aspect is a detailed description of the doctor's entire scope of practice. In recent years, the emergence of portfolio careers means that any appraiser has to be aware of the "other" roles that doctors can develop in addition to their clinical work. The flex-ibility potentially afforded by a portfolio career can help to establish a better work–life balance, giving opportunity for family life and also a help in preparing for retirement (Handy 1991). It is important, however, that the doctor applies proportionate focus on each portfolio and in par-ticular on all clinical roles.

3 On reviewing the content of any reflection it is important to note if the doctor has been clear about their involvement. A significant amount of any doctor's activity is undertaken in the context of a team. The appraiser must make sure that the doctor is clearly stating their contribution, and if this is not the case then it is a question to note for the face-to-face appraisal meeting.

4 Whist reading through the documentation the appraiser has to make a judgment as to the level of reflection shown by the appraisee. Also, there is a need to identify any action that they might want to take or have already taken – what they have learnt and how they are applying that learning in new and different contexts. This theme of personal professional development is essential.

5 Any supporting information should be available and relevant with clear evidence of the doctor reflecting.

6 The exact annual and five-yearly requirements across each of the four countries in the UK do vary, but a common theme is the need for the doctor to provide evidence of reflection across the four domains for appraisal and assessment. There is also a need for 360° feedback from patients and colleagues.

7 It is important that there is evidence of the doctor reflecting on their achievements and strengths over the appraisal period and not just reflecting on issues or constraints.

8 It is important to look at progress on last year's Personal Development Plan (PDP) and any reflections the appraisee has provided on constraints or barriers that delayed or prevented progress.

9 On reviewing the SI it is important to check that no patients or colleagues are, or could be, identified. If patients are identifiable, there must be evidence of consent from the patients. It is acceptable to name colleagues on any published work.

10 The issue of reflecting on near-misses or deaths of patients has been the focus of much media attention. The case of Jack Adcock, a six-year-old boy who died from sepsis in 2011, has had far-reaching consequences across health and particularly in medicine. Jack, who had Down's syndrome, was admitted to Leicester Royal Infirmary with vomiting and diarrhea, but died 11 hours later following unsuccessful resuscitation.

In December 2015 Dr Hadiza Bawa-Garba, a pediatric trainee, and a nurse Isabel Amaro were both convicted of gross negligence manslaughter (GNM) and given a two-year jail term suspended for two years.

One concern is that prior to February 2018 there was a misunderstanding in the general public, and particularly amongst doctors in training, that the High Court had subpoenaed elements of the trainee's e-portfolio where she had reflected on the Adcock case, and that these reflective entries in her e-portfolio had a material effect on the High Court ruling. It became clear following the Medical Protection statement (Medical Protection 2018) that the e-portfolio was not subpoenaed by the Court. Indeed, the Court was clear that reflections were irrelevant to the facts to be determined and that no weight should be given to remarks documented after the event.

As a result of the media and public interest, a rapid review of the application of GNM in the NHS was undertaken (Williams 2018). A key recommendation was that there should be a change in legislation to prevent the GMC and the General Optic Council (GOC) from requiring information from registrants for fitness-to-practice purposes from their reflective practice material. This in effect now gives reflections in appraisals and on e-portfolios (for doctors in training) legal protection.

11 As the appraiser, a useful technique is to identify two or three areas that you would want to explore in more depth in the meeting and suggest to the doctor for them to do likewise. This can help to focus the discussion at least in the earlier stages of the meeting. These points do not need to be strictly adhered to, as they may trigger discussions about more important (to the appraisee) areas.

12 By going through the documentation it can be useful to make notes of key areas, gaps, inconsistencies or any imbalance of focus so that you can explore or give feedback on these in the meeting. If there are significant gaps or inadequate detail, then it can be appropriate to recommend to the doctor that the appraisal meeting is delayed in order to give them time to complete any gaps.

Activities in the Meeting

There are no hard and fast rules about how to conduct an appraisal meeting. However, a key point to remember is that this is the appraisee's appraisal, and as such it is important that you focus on what they want to get out of it. As the appraiser there are, however, a number of key functions that you will have to undertake detailed below.

1 **The environment**
2 **Setting the scene**
3 **Review of last year's PDP**
4 **Discussion of the supporting information**
5 **Agreeing relevant material**
6 **Discussion of any constraints**
7 **Agreeing the provisional PDP for the next year**
8 **Concluding the meeting**

The Environment

It is important to set the right conditions conducive to a confidential meeting. If possible, it is best not to hold the meeting in a busy clinical area or in a room where staff will interrupt. Consider an appropriate off-site venue if that suits the appraisee. Staff should be aware that the meeting must not be interrupted. Get the basics right. Whenever possible have a room that is adequately heated, well lit, with a desk or table with chairs. Turn all phones off and put them away to reduce the temptation to check. As the appraiser you must ensure that adequate time has been set aside by you and by the doctor to allow in-depth and meaningful discussion.

Setting the Scene
At the beginning of the appraisal meeting it is useful for the appraiser to introduce themselves if they have not previously met the appraisee. The appraiser should set the scene of the meeting, explaining the purpose, and share with the appraisee how they wish to proceed. It is useful to check with the doctor if there are any pressing new issues that they have not had a chance to include formally in the SI that they now wish to discuss.

The appraiser should also agree practical issues such as length of the meeting, comfort breaks, and if they plan to take notes throughout the meeting. It is important all of these are discussed in an open manner so that the appraisee feels comfortable with the process.

Review of Last Year's PDP
A useful starting point is reviewing the outcomes from the last PDP. It is not uncommon that the doctor may not have completed all planned objectives. Exploration of those areas completed can help steer further reflection on whether this learning led to new learning needs. Discussion of the reasons for partial or non-completion should be recorded. These can help identify the constraints and challenges that the appraisee has had to face. Early identification of these can help steer discussions.

If there are any objectives not achieved, it is important to discuss whether the appraisee feels they are still relevant and could be rolled into this year's PDP. It is important that the appraiser should be non-judgmental and simply record the reasons as discussed by the doctor.

Discussion of the Supporting Information
Discussion of the appraisal material usually takes up most of the appraisal session and is linked to the learning that they had experienced in the PDP areas. There is no hard and fast rule with regard to the sequence of discussion of SI. One approach is to ask the appraisee to reflect on any achievements they are proud of. This can help to set a positive atmosphere at the beginning of the meeting and help put the appraisee at ease.

It is important to encourage the appraisee to reflect on what they have learnt and how they have used the new learning and or how they plan to use it. This is essentially Kolb's cycle in action (Kolb 1984), discussed in more detail in Chapter 5.

Agreeing Relevant Material

The GMC has been very clear with regard to the types of SI that should be used. A part of the appraiser role is to broker an agreement with the appraisee on the SI that would be most beneficial for the appraisee to discuss. Although CPD credits from a range of organizations may be recorded and discussed, the GMC is clear that this is not an essential requirement. It is important to remember that any of the six types of SI that have been submitted can be discussed in depth.

Discussion of any Constraints

Any constraints and challenges may have already been flagged when reviewing any of last year's PDP objectives that have not been completed. If not, the appraiser should specifically raise this and allow the doctor to reflect on any that might be relevant.

It is useful to get an understanding of what action the doctor has taken to mitigate any constraints and to what extent they have been supported by their employer. A deeper understanding can help the appraiser to put any new PDP objectives in context and assess how realistic and feasible they are. These need to be recorded by the appraiser.

Agreeing the Provisional PDP for Next Year

The role of the appraiser is not to decide on the PDP for the appraisee. The role is to facilitate discussion that allows the appraisee to reflect and come to a decision on what learning objectives would best suit their needs. A good outcome is when the doctor feels an ownership of the PDP, as they are more likely to achieve the stated objectives.

Facilitating a PDP that will be useful and effective for the doctor is an important part of the appraisal. Most doctors will not benefit from a rigid PDP. After the appraisal, more pressing educational or clinical needs may arise which supersede the agreed objectives in the PDP. Many doctors also prefer to learn more spontaneously, making use of opportunities as they occur. If the doctor prefers to learn opportunistically, this can be written into their PDP. It is important to stress that the PDP is flexible, but it will provide a starting point for the next year's appraisal, and should be used by the doctor to structure their planned learning over the following year.

Potential areas for the PDP for next year may have been identified in a number of ways:

1 As stated above, a frequent starting point are any CPD aims that the appraisee was not able to complete from the last appraisal. One issue in this scenario is to check that the learning needs are still relevant.

2 The doctor may have identified learning that they wish to undertake but from the evidence provided this does not appear to link to their role. Sometimes the appraisee will identify aspirational learning . . . the ideal, but any learning objective should map to their scope of practice.

3 Another common driver for revised learning needs is a change in role. For example, if the appraisee had just taken up a formal education role in a medical school, then learning mapped to this role is appropriate and would be expected. Sometimes the appraisee does not know that they do not know, the "unconscious incompetent" (Curtiss and Warren 1974), and a part of the face-to-face discussion may be signposting them to sources of specialist advice regarding meeting any unmet learning needs.

4 The doctor may have identified learning needs through a range of tools such as CPD peer support groups, service change, audit or following discussion with their mentor. These and other tools are explored in detail in Chapter 5.

5 It can happen that new learning objectives are identified through the discussion that the appraisee had not considered previously. You should remember that the doctor needs to "own" their PDP. If you, as the appraiser, are too directive in your approach to the PDP, the doctor is unlikely to engage with it.

Ideally the PDP should:

- Record a small number of agreed specific areas that the appraisee will focus on – these will need to be realistic and achievable within the agreed timeframe
- Avoid generating a long list of development areas across all of the SI
- Include learning that can occur informally and not necessarily require a formal course or taught program – opportunistic learning should be encouraged and a lot of doctors will prefer this type of learning
- Incorporate a level of flexibility so that it can be altered if needed.

Concluding the Meeting

Many doctors find the whole process of appraisal stressful, and it is likely that the discussion will have been intense and wide-ranging. It is therefore useful to try and summarize the main points. Certainly it is of value to reiterate the PDP and also give the opportunity for the doctor to feed back to the appraiser.

Action Post-meeting

A key role for the appraiser is to prepare a summary of key discussions that took place in the appraisal meeting. Again, the exact format for this will vary across the four UK nations and within regions, but there are key principles. These include the following:

- Record a summary of each discussion you had with the appraisee. This should be objective and not include any value judgments. Summarize each discussion under headings such as:
  - a description of the event/situation
  - the reason the appraisee chose this and the potential impact
  - any reflections that the appraisee offered
  - action taken or being planned to be taken by the appraisee.
- Ensure the summary is an accurate reflection of the discussion. If you have any concerns at the meeting, there is always the option of meeting again and suggesting to the appraisee what areas need more clarification or additional SI before submitting or finalizing the summary. It is important to remember that the summary is used by the RO to enable them to make a recommendation to the GMC.

Skills Required of a Good Appraiser

Good communication skills are essential for facilitating the appraisal and the process of identifying key areas for the appraisee. If the appraisal is to be meaningful and hence fit for purpose, there are a number of key skills required of the appraiser in the meeting:

a **Active listening**
b **Providing feedback**
c **Coaching skills**

These areas are interlinked, but for completeness each will be discussed in detail below.

Active Listening

As an appraiser, developing the skills of an active listener are vital. This is highly important in the context of an appraisal in order to set the conditions to provide a safe space for genuine and honest reflection. Active listening means paying full attention to the person as they are talking to you. This is different to the passive hearing that we do on a day-to-day basis. It entails giving the person your full attention. A key element is showing the other person that you are truly listening to them. It is about being as fully present in the moment as possible.

Active listening is important for a number of reasons. When someone sees that you are actively listening, they are more likely to believe that you care about what they are saying. When you are showing someone that you are very interested in what they are saying, they will tend to feel that you are trying to understand them. Practicing active listening means that you are more likely to catch more details and important nuances you might otherwise miss, and thus avoid misunderstandings.

There are a number of key steps to being an active listener. The following are a number of key techniques that can be used to improve active listening skills, and we will explore each:

1 **Be aware of your own body language**
2 **Control your internal voice**
3 **Be aware of the appraisee's body language**
4 **Verbal interaction**
5 **Open-ended questions**
6 **Probing questions**
7 **Paraphrasing**
8 **Reflection**
9 **Neutral techniques**
10 **Summarizing**

Be Aware of Your Body Language

It is important to be aware of your body language and to manage the environment by reducing access to any potential distractions. Remove items from the area if they are not needed, thus reducing the risk of you flicking a pen, checking your mobile or looking around the room. Appearing restless or fidgety gives the impression that you are not interested in what the other person is saying.

If the person with whom you are engaging in conversation is sitting back, cross-legged, with arms folded in their lap, it is useful on occasions to mirror a similar image in your own body language. This will subconsciously indicate to them that you are listening to them, and will put their mind at ease, facilitating more open and honest discussion.

It is important to maintain regular eye contact with the other person. When you do this you are forced to pay attention to that person and you will be less likely to be distracted. This technique also conveys a powerful message to the other person that you are treating the interaction as important. This is a vital message to allow trust to build up.

Listeners need to confirm that they are following the flow of conversation by placing nods of confirmation at the appropriate cues in the conversation. Developing active listening skills utilizes this body language to great effect, allowing speakers to continue talking without disrupting their communication flow.

Control Your Internal Voice

Everyone has an internal voice, or internal monolog, that you "hear" inside your head. This internal voice can be useful in helping to plan and problem-solve, but in the context of a high-stakes meeting such as an appraisal, it is important that the internal voice does not act as a distraction.

Be Aware of the Appraisee's Body Language

It is important to be aware of the nonverbal clues that the other person is giving off while speaking. If they are uncomfortable, they might fidget. If they are nervous, they may avoid looking directly at you. These types of nonverbal clues can help you focus on how the other person is feeling. You can pick up a lot of what a person is communicating to you through their body language and not the actual words used.

Verbal Interaction

The art of active listening could be characterized by the appraiser speaking less, which gives the appraisee the greatest opportunity to develop their own thoughts as well as ideas. This principle of limiting your interrupting is not a hard and fast rule, as you will sometimes need to ask questions, but it is vital to remember that it is the appraisee's appraisal.

Aiming for minimal talking is a good objective, but at certain points in the meeting you will need to question the appraisee. There are a number of types of question to focus on.

Open-ended Questions

If the appraisee hesitates or is finding it difficult to articulate, do use open-ended questions to gather more information. It is best to avoid closed questions that lead to YES/NO answers, such as . . . "is that a problem for you?"

When someone has a hard time getting through everything, it's okay to provide some light encouragement here and there to get them to continue speaking or share more details.

You do not want to rush into it, but when the appraisee seems to be in the middle of exploring an event or incident and comes to a halt, you can say something short like:

> *And then. . .?*
> *What happened next?*
> *Anything else?*
> *What do think about that?*
> *How do you feel about what happened?*
> *How did it affect you?*
> *What impact did that have on other members of the team?*

Probing Questions

At certain points in the meeting it is appropriate to probe for more information when needed. Remember that your goal is not to take over the conversation – it is to actively listen to the other person. Now when you feel there could be more relevant information that has not come out yet, it is appropriate to ask a few probing questions.

Asking things such as, "how did that make you feel?" or "what do you think is the best way to handle that situation?" are good ways to get the other person to share more about how they feel. This helps you understand the situation better.

There are a number of other key verbal techniques that will help in the appraisal process/interaction. According to Newkirk and Linden (1982) some of these techniques are: *paraphrasing, reflection, neutral techniques* and *summarizing.*

Paraphrasing

Paraphrasing is when the listener restates in their own words what the speaker means. This is valuable in testing the understanding of what the speaker means and lets them know you are paying attention. There are risks in paraphrasing, as it can be perceived as if the appraiser is second-guessing the speaker's next words. Another risk is that it can be perceived as the appraiser trying to speed up the conversation.

Recap what is said to you. When the appraisee is reflecting on an incident that is clearly important to them, it is useful to repeat what they have said. This will not only show them you were listening, but it will also ensure that you remember what was said to you later. Again, one way to ensure you have heard them is to say something like: "So, if I understand you correctly, you want. . .(insert what they have just said to you here)." This will keep both you and the speaker on track and focused on the conversation.

If you are in any doubt about what the appraisee is saying/meaning, ask clarifying questions. Do not criticize them, but ask questions that will show that you are paying attention and are truly interested in the topic they are discussing.

Reflection

Reflection is slightly different from paraphrasing; here the listener tells the speaker what they believe their feelings are rather than the content of the message. This is particularly important when the speaker expresses strong feelings. This active feedback loop has the effect of reconfirming to the appraisee that you have understood everything they have said.

Neutral Techniques

Neutral techniques encourage the speaker to continue talking. A simple nod of the head or a "uh-huh" are usually effective signals that the listener is interested and listening.

Summarizing

Summarizing involves combining the speaker's thoughts into a concise statement that focuses on the speaker's key points. This is a particularly useful technique to help sense-check that the appraiser has understood what has been discussed.

Providing Feedback

The appraisal meeting is a key element in medical revalidation, and a role of the appraiser is to ensure that there is a robustness to the process. A routine task is to provide the appraisee with feedback on a number of things:

- The level of detail in the SI
- The type of SI and its appropriateness
- The balance of the SI
- The appraisee's level of engagement in genuine reflection
- The appraisee's ability and keenness to engage in learning, and as a result change their behavior
- The appropriateness of the proposed PDP.

It is clear that the skills to provide feedback in a constructive manner are essential. The timing, focus and appropriate level of feedback along with constructive challenge will be decided by the appraiser, taking cues from the appraisee. The appraisee, through the process of the appraisal discussion, may engage in "self-challenge."

Feedback can be seen as potentially threatening by both the appraisee and the appraiser. As the person giving feedback, you may fear that the relationship will be affected by the process, especially if there is an element of poor performance that needs to be addressed. The appraisee, as the receiver of feedback, can sometimes react negatively, becoming defensive or angry. So the idea of setting a framework for feedback at the outset of the relationship can be useful.

Pendleton et al. (1984) developed a set of guidelines to help structure feedback. Using this model, the process entails the giver of feedback firstly focusing on what the individual has done well, the positive aspects. After this the focus is on what could have been done better. However, this approach has been criticized as being possibly too simplistic and formulaic, with the risk that the receivers of the feedback focus too much on the negative aspects.

Silverman et al. (2013) have described a framework for giving feedback. The model is based on an agenda-led approach with analysis of the proposed outcomes. The first task for the appraiser is to clarify the appraisee's agenda and explore with them any difficulties or challenges they have experienced and what help they would like. The next step is to explore the appraisee's proposed outcomes and encourage them to reflect on a number of possible solutions to the challenges.

With all feedback there is need for the appraiser to avoid being judgmental and maintain an objective stance. The aim is to enable the appraisee to recognize any areas for improvement but also acknowledge for themselves areas of good practice.

There are a number of skills that can enable one to challenge in a constructive way that helps the appraisee. Challenging should always be done with empathy, so it is important that appraisers avoid challenging to meet their own personal needs, instead of the appraisee's. Some of the techniques include:

1 **Immediacy**
2 **Self-disclosure**
3 **Reframing**
4 **Metaphors**

Immediacy

Immediacy is a useful technique to help focus the appraisee on the here and now within the session, helping to increase the individual's self-awareness (Teyber 2006). Process comments are one form of immediacy that involve the appraiser cueing the appraisee to focus on the interpersonal process in the session rather than the session content.

For example, the appraiser might say, "When I just shared my view of what you were saying, I noticed your facial expression changed. I'm wondering what you were you feeling as I said that to you." This can help the appraisee to focus on the immediate interaction and gain a level of conscious insight that can then enable reflection.

In addition, the appraiser may share how what was said or the way it was said affected them. This is a form of self-disclosure by the appraiser (Kelly 2017). This is a technique used in a variety of counseling models, but is extremely effective as a means to challenge defensiveness.

Self-Disclosure

Self-disclosure was mentioned above. This is a tool we all use to some extent in our day-to-day interactions with each other, in both professional and personal situations. It is simply the appraiser providing information about themselves. This general social skill is used to build bonds. In the context of an appraisal it can be useful for the appraiser to engage in some level of self-disclosure, but one needs to be careful not to over-use this technique. If this happens the appraisal can start to feel as if it is about you, the appraiser. This will have the effect of disengaging the appraisee from the process. It is important to use this approach sparingly and for a specific purpose in the meeting. There is also a risk that, if overused, you project a false image of only sharing the good information about you. This again can have a detrimental effect on the appraisee's perception of your role.

Reframing

Reframing is a skill that is grounded in cognitive therapy and is used to help the appraisee to see a situation or problem in a different, often more positive, light. The essential idea behind reframing is that a person's point of view depends upon the frame in which it is viewed. When the frame is shifted, the meaning changes and thinking and behavior often change along with it.

Reframing often involves recognizing the individual's positive intentions and communicating an understanding that they are doing the best that they can, given the constraints and pressures that they are facing.

The issues for an appraisee can be broadly external ("my Clinical Director doesn't understand what I need to do") or internal ("I should be further on in my career by now"). Helping them to see these issues from a different angle can enable them to find solutions themselves.

Metaphors

It is useful for the appraiser to listen out for the appraisee using metaphors. These are typically used to share complex, difficult-to-grasp experiences. A metaphor is stating one thing is something else that is completely unrelated. These can be explored to gain understanding and empathy. The appraiser can also use metaphors to challenge the appraisee to think about an idea in a new way or to take a different perspective.

Some metaphors to look out for include:

> *his students are puppets on a string*
> *there is a blanket of secrecy over the changes in the protocol for. . .*
> *the trainee's mind is a sponge*

Coaching Skills

There are a number of coaching methods that can be used in an appraisal setting to help the appraiser firstly to formulate the issue/concern/opportunity themselves, to then be able to facilitate the appraisee in being able to identify their own solutions.

One model that is widely used in medicine and across a wide range of sectors is the GROW model (Whitmore 2009), based in large part on the Inner Game model (Gallwey 1974). We will explore this model in detail and also describe a hybrid version called ACHIEVE (Dembkowski and Eldridge 2003). Both will be compared and contrasted, and it is important to note that both approaches are equally valid and appropriate methods that can help you structure the discussion around specific issues.

The GROW model

GROW stands for:

- Goal
- Current Reality
- Options (or obstacles)
- Will (or the way forward)

This model can assist the appraiser in facilitating the discussion to help the appraisee to identify their own solutions or action plans. One of the benefits of this approach is that it is a generic one, which enables the individual to develop and maintain ownership of their own solutions, meaning that they are more likely to achieve them. Therefore, it is important at the end of the process that the appraisee has a sense of ownership of the action plan, the PDP.

It is important to note that the GROW model assumes that the coach (appraiser in this case) is not necessarily an expert in the appraisee's field. This means that the appraiser acts as a facilitator, helping the appraisee to select the best options.

In this role with this model, the appraiser is not there to offer advice, guidance or their personal opinion on what they would do or have done in a similar situation. It is more empowering for the appraisee to come to their own conclusions.

To structure a coaching or mentoring session using the GROW Model, take the following steps:

1 What is the **Goal**?
  The first step is to enable the appraisee to be clear about their goal. What is it they want to achieve? It is vital that the goal is SMART, one that is:
  - Specific
  - Measurable
  - Attainable
  - Realistic
  - Time-bound

To get to this point, posing questions such as the following can help the appraisee to frame their goal:

How will you know that you have achieved this goal?

How will others, members of your team, know?

How will you know if the issue has been resolved?

2 Explore the current **Reality**

The next step is to get the appraisee to explore their current position, their current reality. This is a key step, because if the individual is not aware of their starting point on this journey, it will be difficult for them to decide any actions they need to take or consider. They may make erroneous assumptions or ignore information that is required to get them where they want to be. As the appraisee starts to explore their current reality, solutions frequently start to emerge.

Useful coaching questions in this step include the following:

- What is happening now (what, who, when, and how often)? What is the effect or result of this?
- Have you already taken any steps toward your goal?
- Does this goal conflict with any other goals or objectives?

3 Explore the **Options**

The next step is to enable the individual to explore what options, in reality, are open to them. It is best to allow the individual, at least in the beginning, to explore all possible options before helping them to focus on those that are realistic. This may require challenging the appraisee. Then, discuss these and help them decide on the best ones.

It is important in this stage to ensure you do not generate the options yourself, but let the appraisee reflect on what is possible. The role of the appraiser in this model is to guide the individual in the right direction, without actually making decisions for them.

Again, the use of the following open questions can be useful:

- What else could you do?
- What if this, or that constraint, were removed? Would that change things?
- What are the advantages and disadvantages of each option?
- What factors or considerations will you use to weigh the options?
- What do you need to stop doing in order to achieve this goal?
- What obstacles stand in your way?

4 Establish the **Will** (or **Way** forward)

The way forward frequently follows from the discussions of the reality and options. The final step is to enable the appraisee to commit to a series of actions, the PDP, to move toward the goal. Useful questions to ask here include:

- So, what will you do now, and when? What else will you do?
- What could stop you moving forward? How will you overcome this?
- How can you keep yourself motivated?
- When do you need to review progress? Daily, weekly, monthly?

ACHIEVE

The other model to consider is ACHIEVE (Dembkowski and Eldridge 2003). It is argued that its advantage over the GROW model is in providing more flexibility and feedback-reactivity. One of the aims of this model is to increase trust between the appraisee and the appraiser, and increase understanding of the methods involved in goal-setting and problem-solving.

The seven stages of the ACHIEVE model are:
- Assess the current situation
- Creative brainstorming
- Hone goals
- Initiate option generation
- Evaluate options
- Valid action program design
- Encourage momentum.

1 Assess the current situation

This is similar to the exploring reality stage in the GROW model, where the appraisee is encouraged to reflect on their current situation. This can help the individual have a greater understanding as to how certain situations have arisen, enabling identification of appropriate solutions. There is, however, more of an emphasis on the appraisee reflecting on how they triggered emotional reactions and responses in others, adding a layer of emotional intelligence (Goleman 1995).

2 Creative brainstorming

This stage is designed to unlock the appraisee's thinking and help them move away from repeated behavior that has not been constructive. When under any form of pressure or stress, we all have a tendency to narrow down our thinking to a binary position (Joseph and Newman 2010). Brainstorming is a useful tool to facilitate creative problem-solving and can be used one-to-one or in small groups (Osborn 1963). In practice, pose a question to the individual and get them to offer up any possible solutions, in a free-flowing way. Brainstorming works best if some principles are adhered to;
- Go for quantity . . . the more ideas the more chance of finding the best solution
- No criticism . . . no judgments should be made on any ideas offered
- Encourage wild ideas . . . these may stimulate further new ideas.

3 Hone goals

In this stage the appraisee develops goals from the range of ideas generated in the previous step. As with the GROW model, any solutions need to be SMART. These goals are revised and refined with the appraiser.

4 Initiate option generation

At this stage in the process, the immediate steps to achieve the goals are considered. The aim is to facilitate the appraisee to develop a wide range of options, and not at this point focus on the feasibility of any, or focus on what s/he believes is the single right one.

5 Evaluate options

After generating a number of options the appraisee is guided to evaluate each one and start to prioritize. It is vital that any aims are well defined so that the steps to achieving them are clear and achievable. As the appraiser your role is to help the individual focus on a smaller number of feasible aims.

6 Valid action programme design

The aim of this stage is for the appraisee to put the options into action. A good way of encouraging this is for the appraisee to split each aim down into smaller steps, with clear action points and deadlines. The key element is the individual committing to the plan, and as they work through the steps to generalize any learning to other situations and scenarios.

7 Encourage momentum

The key role of the appraiser at this stage is to encourage the appraisee by recognizing and praising when steps are taken, however small. The complexity of issues that may arise frequently mean that the individual has to take a number of steps over a period of time in order to achieve the goal. There is a real risk that motivation and confidence will be dented leading to loss of focus and ultimately not achieving the goal. It is important that any small steps achieved are celebrated.

Repeat

The ACHIEVE process is flexible and repetitive. Once any goal has been achieved or even partially achieved, then the process can be applied again, since as a result of action taken, the situation and environment will most likely have changed.

In summary, GROW and ACHIEVE are two associated models that any appraiser can use depending on the nature of the working relationship with the appraisee.

The Role of the Responsible Officer (RO)

The Responsible Officer (RO) role was introduced and their responsibilities set out under the Medical Profession (Responsible Officers) Regulations 2010. The legislation sets out that the RO should be appointed or nominated by a DB as set out in the Medical Act 1983 (as amended by the Health and Social Care Act 2008). The detailed roles and responsibilities are set out in guidance updated in July 2010 (Department of Health 2010). The key areas that apply to ROs in England, Scotland and Wales are summarized below.

- The ROs are senior doctors with a GMC license to practice and, at the time of appointment, they must have been a fully registered medical practitioner for the previous five years.
- ROs are charged with ensuring that all doctors with a connection to their organization (the DB) work within a managed environment in which their performance, conduct and behavior are monitored against agreed national standards.
- If there are concerns about a doctor's fitness to practice, the ROs have the authority and responsibility to instigate investigation of the doctor's performance and to ensure that the appropriate action is taken.
- If the cause of concern is found to relate to the systems in which the doctor is working rather than an individual doctor, the RO has a duty to ensure that the DB takes action to address any issues.

Although some aspects of the role can be delegated to others, it is the RO that personally makes a recommendation to the GMC. On a five-yearly cycle each RO can make one of three possible recommendations about an individual doctor. These are:

1 A positive recommendation that the doctor is up to date, fit to practice and should be revalidated.
2 Request a deferral because they need more information to make a recommendation about the doctor.
3 Notify the GMC that the doctor has failed to engage with any of the local systems or processes (such as appraisal) that support revalidation.

The medical revalidation process sits alongside fitness-to-practice procedures. The regulations state explicitly that if at any point in the five-year cycle an RO has concerns that a doctor is not fit to practice, they should refer the doctor into the GMC's fitness-to-practice process. The RO must not wait until a revalidation recommendation is due.

The RO is charged with specific actions which include:

- Systems for collecting and holding information that informs fitness-to-practice decisions

- To ensure there are rigorous appraisal processes in place
- To ensure there is an integrated system for monitoring doctors' performance
- Identifying at an early stage if there are any fitness to practice issues and taking appropriate action
- Encouraging a learning and development culture
- Ensuring that the organization is informed of the resources required to support the systems, data collection, appraisal and CPD
- Liaising with the GMC on matters linked to fitness-to-practice issues.

It is the responsibility of the RO to ensure there are procedures in place to monitor the compliance of any doctor whose practice is supervised and/or limited under conditions imposed by, or undertakings given to, the GMC.

As all ROs are doctors with a licence to practice, they too must have an RO. The operation of these higher ROs varies across the UK. In England, the RO at a local level will relate to a RO at the appropriate Strategic Health Authority, and in Scotland and Wales the ROs of local responsible officers will be based within the Scottish and Welsh Governments respectively.

These RO regulations apply to all ROs in England, Scotland and Wales. The details of supporting processes do vary from organization to organization.

There is a range of support for ROs such as the Employer Liaison Adviser (ELA) role, a GMC role established to be a link with the regulator and to help advise ROs regarding thresholds for referral into the GMC and general advice regarding benchmarking of decisions. Typically, ELAs work across a number of ROs and are seen as a valuable resource.

The Designated Body (DB)

The role of the DB is set out in GMC guidance. For most doctors their DB will be their main employer. Across the UK these range from large NHS trusts to private hospitals and locum agencies. All doctors must have a connection to a DB in order to revalidate.

The responsibilities of DBs are:

- to appoint a RO to support the process of revalidation
- to support ROs through a range of resources for them to be able to discharge their roles as detailed above
- to ensure there are an adequate number of appropriately trained appraisers in post or available
- to establish, maintain and develop IT and other systems which support doctors to collect SI
- to enable all doctors employed by the DB to be able to identify their DB

- to have systems in place so that all doctors with a connection can record their revalidation date and allow ROs to make timely recommendations
- to provide and signpost to a range of resources to support doctors in appraisal and revalidation
- to have systems in place to easily share information potentially useful for appraisal, such as complaints, compliments and feedback
- to have an up-to-date appraisal system that makes sure every licensed doctor is having a regular appraisal
- to ensure fully functioning clinical governance systems that can provide doctors with the SI they need for appraisal and revalidation
- implement policies and systems to identify and respond to concerns about doctors
- have robust links with the other organizations where doctors may also be working, so information about their practice and any concerns about them can be shared.

Requirements for Doctors in Training

Doctors in training revalidate by being actively engaged in all aspects of the requirement of their relevant training program.

This means each doctor in training must:

- engage in and meet the assessment and other requirements of the training program
- discuss progress and learning needs with the educational supervisors
- declare any practice undertaken outside of the training program, for example, locums must be disclosed and discussed.

The RO for doctors in training varies across the UK. In Scotland and Wales the RO is the Medical Director of the respective statutory medical education bodies: NHS Education Scotland, and Health Education and Improvement Wales. In Northern Ireland the RO is the Postgraduate Medical Dean, and in England the Regional Deans (or equivalents).

As with other doctors, the ROs will usually make a revalidation recommendation to the GMC every five years. The recommendation is based on the doctor's active participation in the Annual Review of Competence Progression (ARCP) process, or equivalent. The ARCP is considered equivalent to the appraisal that all other doctors are required to engage in. In addition, doctors in training are not required to gather and submit SI. For ARCPs, meeting the requirements of the training program is seen as equivalent.

Any work outside of the training program must be declared on Form R as a part of the ARCP process. Completion of Form R (Part B) is an important element of the ARCP which allows the RO to be assured that the doctor in training is engaged with their training and there are no fitness-to-practice issues declared. The members of the ARCP panel are likely to have information from, for example, the Educational Supervisor report and other sources that can verify or otherwise any declaration on the form.

Form R is a self-declaration confirming the following:

1 Whole scope of practice, including locums or private work. Any voluntary work is best declared if in any doubt.
2 That the doctor accepts the professional obligations placed on them with regard to honesty and integrity as stated in GMP.
3 That they accept the professional obligations placed on them with regard to their personal health in GMP.
4 A declaration if the doctor has any GMC conditions, warnings or undertakings placed on them by the GMC, employing Trust or any other organization.
5 If the doctor is subject to any conditions they have to declare that they are complying with such conditions or undertakings.
6 A section that allows the doctor on a voluntary basis to declare anything in relation to their health, if they feel that it would be beneficial for the ARCP panel or RO to be aware of.
7 If any previous Significant Events, Complaints or Other Investigations were declared, to comment on their status and that the doctor has reflected on these in the portfolio.
8 If any previously declared Significant Events, Complaints or Other Investigations remain unresolved. If this is the case, the doctor should provide a summary and their reflections.
9 The option of detailing any voluntary work and to include any positive feedback and/or compliments

In summary, the process for doctors in training is different to other doctors. The key requirement is to show that they are actively engaged with the training program, the ARCP and associated documentation, as this is seen as equivalent to the appraisal process for other doctors.

Chapter Summary

In this chapter we have considered the roles and responsibilities of three key players in medical revalidation: the appraiser, the RO, and the DB.

We have summarized the four GMC domains and the SI that should be used in the appraisal process as set out by the GMC. In regard to appraisal of GPs, SAS doctors and Consultants, we have explored tasks before the meeting, during the meeting and after the appraisal meeting. Within the meeting we have touched on a number of areas including the environment, a review of last year's PDP, discussion of the SI and any constraints, and an agreed PDP for the next year.

We have emphasized the importance of the summary document being an accurate reflection of the discussion and objectives, as this is the main source of evidence generally used by ROs to make recommendations.

We have considered the skills required to perform as a good appraiser, including active listening skills, the ability and confidence to challenge constructively, provide feedback, and coaching skills that can be used.

We have summarized the roles and responsibilities of the RO and designated bodies as set in law, and have also detailed the process for doctors in training to successfully revalidate.

References

Curtiss, P.R. and Warren, P.W. (1974). *The Dynamics of Life Skills Coaching. Life Skills Series*. Prince Albert, Saskatchewan: Training Research and Development Station, Dept. of Manpower and Immigration.

Dembkowski, S. and Eldridge, F. (2003). Beyond GROW: a new coaching model. *International Journal of Mentoring and Coaching* **1** (1).

Department of Health (2010). *Medical regulation: responsible officer guidance*. https://www.gov.uk/government/publications/closing-the-gap-in-medical-regulation-responsible-officer-guidance (accessed 8 May 2021).

Gallwey, W.T. (1974). *The Inner Game of Tennis*. New York: Random House.

General Medical Council (2017). *Generic professional capabilities framework*. Manchester: General Medical Council. https://www.gmc-uk.org/education/standards-guidance-and-curricula/standards-and-outcomes/generic-professional-capabilities-framework (accessed 8 May 2021).

General Medical Council (2020). *Guidance on Supporting Information for Appraisal and Revalidation*. London: GMC.

Goleman, D.J. (1995). *Emotional Intelligence: Why it Can Matter More than IQ*. London: Bloomsbury Publishing.

Handy, C. (1991). The Age of Unreason. Harvard Business Review Press.

Joseph, D.L. and Newman, D.A. (2010). Emotional intelligence: an integrated meta-analysis and cascading model. *Journal of Applied Psychology* **95**: 54–78.

Kelly, K. (2017). *Basic Counselling Skills: A Student Guide*. Counsellor Tutor Ltd.

Kolb, D.A. (1984). *Experiential Learning Experience as a Source of Learning and Development*. New Jersey: Prentice Hall.

Medical Protection (2018). E-portfolios and the Dr Bawa-Garba case – Dr Pallavi Bradshawclarifies.https://www.medicalprotection.org/uk/articles/e-portfolios-and-the-dr-bawa-garba-case-dr-pallavi-bradshaw-clarifies (accessed 8 May 2021).

Newkirk, W. and Linden, R. (1982). EMS management: Improving communication through active listening. *Emergency Medical Services* **11**: 8–11.

Nursing and Midwifery Council (2019). Benefits of becoming a reflective practitioner. A joint statement of support from Chief Executives of statutory regulators of health and social care professionals. www.nmc.org.uk/globalassets/sitedocuments/other-publications/benefits-of-becoming-a-reflective-practitioner---joint-statement-2019.pdf (accessed 8 May 2021).

Osborn, A. F. (1963). *Applied Imagination: Principles and Procedures of Creative Problem Solving*, 3e. New York, NY: Charles Scribner's Sons.

Pendleton, D., Scofield, T., Tate, P. et al. (1984). *The Consultation: An Approach to Learning and Teaching*. Oxford: Oxford University Press.

Pype, P., Mertens, F., Helewaut, F. et al. (2018). Healthcare teams as complex adaptive systems: understanding team behaviour through team members' perception of interpersonal interaction. *BMC Health Services Research* **18**: 570. https://doi.org/10.1186/s12913-018-3392-3.

Silverman, J., Kurtz, S., and Draper, J. (2013). *Skills for Communicating with Patients*. Boca Raton, FL: CRC Press.

Teyber, E. (2006). *Interpersonal Process in Therapy: An Integrative Model*. Belmont, CA: Brooks/Cole, Cengage Learning.

UK Medical Revalidation coLLAboration (2018). *Evaluating the regulatory impact of medical revalidation*. https://www.gmc-uk.org/-/media/documents/umbrella-report-final_pdf-74454378.pdf (accessed 8 May 2021).

Whitmore, J. (2009). *Coaching for Performance: GROWing Human Potential and Purpose: The Principle and Practice of Coaching and Leadership. People Skills for Professionals*, 4e. Boston: Nicholas Brealey Publishing.

Williams, N. (2018). *Gross Negligence Manslaughter in Healthcare*. The report of a rapid policy review. https://www.gov.uk/government/publications/williams-review-into-gross-negligence-manslaughter-in-healthcare (accessed 8 May 2021).

Chapter 5 **Revalidation – The Role of the Appraisee**

Introduction

In this chapter we will explore the roles and responsibilities of the appraisee. In particular we will discuss what actions you need to take, in what order, to be able to successfully and meaningfully engage with appraisal. The General Medical Council (GMC 2020a) outlines the values, behaviors and competencies that constitute Good Medical Practice (GMP) in four overarching Domains:

1 **Knowledge, skills and performance**
2 **Safety and quality**
3 **Communication, partnership and teamwork**
4 **Maintaining trust**

Key Principles

The key principles underpinning appraisal are described clearly (GMC 2020a) and summarized under the practical headings of Collect/Reflect/Discuss. The general tasks that are the appraisee's responsibility include:

1 Providing general information that describes the context of all aspects of your work.
2 Providing supporting information (SI) to show that you are keeping up to date and maintaining and enhancing the quality of your professional work.
3 Evidence of you reflecting on your practice, including any feedback from patients and/or colleagues.
4 To include details of your whole scope of practice. If you have a portfolio of roles, for example, half time clinical and half medical management, there is a need to reflect on both roles and provide SI that covers all aspects.

How to Succeed at Revalidation, First Edition. Peter Donnelly and Katie Webb.
© 2022 John Wiley & Sons Ltd. Published 2022 by John Wiley & Sons Ltd.

These may also include voluntary activities, postgraduate training, under-graduate teaching or academic roles that are not necessarily directly patient-facing.

5 It is important to remember that it is not about the quantity of your reflections but rather the quality. The GMC does not set a minimum or maximum number of SIs that you must collect.

6 Your SI must be proportional. It is best to choose key examples that allow the generation of meaningful learning. You should not submit every piece of evidence for each type of SI. Pick the most appropriate.

There are six types of SI you must collect, reflect on and discuss at your appraisal. They are:

a Continuing professional development (CPD)
b Quality improvement activity
c Significant events
d Feedback from patients or those to whom you provide medical services
e Feedback from colleagues
f Compliments and complaints.

Initially we will consider the general principles of how to prepare for appraisal. We will consider the detail of each of these in line with GMC guidance highlighting the following:

1 **Collecting supporting information**
2 **Reflecting on your practice**
3 **Discussing your reflections**
4 **Action you have taken or will be taking.**

Collecting Supporting Information (SI)

It is best, if at all possible to collect information on a continuous basis throughout the year. The focus of your SI can be triggered by any event or experience you have had or witnessed through the appraisal year. It is important to focus equally on positive experiences, compliments and what went well in addition to any untoward incidents. A good starting point is your Personal Development Plan (PDP) from the last appraisal.

Reflect on whether you were able to achieve the objectives, and if not, why not, and what you intend to do or have done to rectify the situation. Reflecting on what you have learned and how you have applied that in practice is important. It is also useful to reflect whether the learning, whatever it was or whatever the format, uncovered other areas of unmet learning needs. These can include:

- clinical events that went well
- achievements
- CPD experiences
- clinical problems
- challenges with patients
- challenges with colleagues
- constraints.

How to Assess Your Own Learning Needs

To get the most out of your appraisal it is important to be aware of your own learning needs. These should take into account your prior learning and any subsequent gaps in knowledge or skills you can identify. This process will ensure any new learning can be focused on meeting your own personal learning needs. This is underpinned by adult learning theory, and once you have identified any gaps in knowledge and or technical skills then you use these to generate an action plan (Knowles et al. 2011). This self-reflection leading to self-assessment of your needs is a key stage in adult learning and is pivotal in any CPD.

When considering any of your learning needs, it is important for you to distinguish between perceived and true learning needs (Laxdal 1982). Self-perceived learning needs are important as they are more likely to be owned by the individual, and this leads in turn to increased motivation and participation. The process leading to identifying one's own perceived learning needs usually entails a mixture of internal and external reflection. The latter, also referred to as informed self-assessment, (Sargeant et al. 2010), is relevant in the appraisal process and one's learning may, in part, be driven by external sources such as changes in clinical guidelines from organizations such as the National Institute for Health and Care Excellence or external standards set out by the GMC.

In the absence of external drivers, there is a risk that the process of self-assessment of perceived needs becomes increasingly subjective. As a result, solely self-assessed perceived needs may not necessarily reflect all that is required.

In comparison, it is argued that true learning needs are objectively generated by external independent assessment of a learner's performance against an agreed standard. This process involves triangulation of information from a wide range of sources, methods, and collection strategies (Lockyer 1998). The sources can include peers, educational supervisors, mentors, and importantly patients. There are of course risks with this external approach because if a learner perceives that learning is imposed on them, they are then less likely to perceive a sense of ownership and personal relevance. This can lead to disengagement in the entire process.

There are a number of useful approaches you can use to identify and generate your own learning needs.

1 **Multi-source feedback – 360° feedback**
2 **Patient-reported outcome measures (PROMs) and patient-reported experience measures (PREMs)**
3 **Peer-to-peer support**
4 **Mentoring/coaching**
5 **The Johari window**
6 **Strengths, weaknesses, opportunities, threats (SWOT) analysis**
7 **Patient's unmet needs (PUNs) and doctor's educational needs (DENs)**
8 **National audits**
9 **Clinical governance processes**
10 **Know yourself – know your learning styles.**

Multi-source Feedback – 360° Feedback
Introduction
Multi-source feedback (MSF) also known as 360° feedback, has been extensively used in a range of organizations and has been widely used in postgraduate training in the UK for a number of years.

The purpose of MSF is articulated on the Scotland medical appraisal website:

> *Colleague Feedback is a process in which colleagues give you feedback on how they perceive you work with them. It looks at a number of attributes applicable to all doctors rather than your individual clinical skills and knowledge. The feedback is usually obtained using an anonymous questionnaire.*
>
> *The purpose of Colleague Feedback (MSF) is to provide you with feedback that gives you an opportunity to reflect on the feedback received and to compare it with your own self-assessment. It is hoped that this will reinforce good practice and provide opportunities for development. The feedback can provide information about important qualities you demonstrate as a doctor, such as integrity, respect and the ability to communicate and work as a team member, and how these are perceived by those you work with.*

(Medical Appraisal Scotland 2021)

The GMC provides example questionnaires to gather patient and colleague feedback. These are designed to be generic and can be used by all doctors irrespective of their specialty or location of clinical practice. There are also examples of questionnaires that can be used (GMC 2021a), if you do not have significant direct face-to-face contact with patients (e.g. public health physicians, microbiologists).

For some doctors who have roles that don't provide patient interaction or work less than full-time or in short-term locums, there are useful case studies on the GMC site (GMC 2021b). One example might be if you only provided medico-legal reports. In this case you are not providing clinical care but providing the courts with a professional opinion on your client. In this scenario it would be appropriate to seek feedback from your clients directly and those other colleagues you interact with, such as solicitors, barristers, and administrative staff, and then reflect on this.

Within the UK the four nations have slightly different supporting processes and infrastructure for appraisal in general and for MSF.

In Scotland there is an online system used in primary care, the Scotland Online Appraise Resource (SOAR), not yet mandatory for those doctors working in secondary care. SOAR allows appraisers and appraisees to share documents and SI online and also allows tracking of the appraisal process. Linked to SOAR is a MSF tool that can be used by appraisees.

In Wales, the Medical Appraisal and Revalidation System (MARS) was first launched in August 2010 by the Wales Deanery, funded by the Welsh Government, initially for GPs only before becoming mandatory for all doctors in Wales (excluding doctors in training) in April 2014. The arguments for the advantages of a single online system include:

- One consistent appraisal system for all doctors
- A single appraisal tool to support Responsible Officers in making their revalidation recommendations
- Consistent opportunities for all doctors
- An automated link to the GMC.

The MARS system transferred to Health Education and Improvement Wales (HEIW) in 2019, and an online MSF tool called ORBIT 360 has been developed and is available to all doctors in Wales.

Examples of Specific MSF Tools

In addition to the GMC questionnaires and those developed by Wales and Scotland, a range of tools have been used and evaluated in certain clinical settings. We will highlight a few examples, but the key issue is that is does not matter which tool is used so long as during the process the following are taken into consideration:

1 Patient confidentiality and anonymity
2 Patients feel comfortable with the process
3 You cannot identify staff or patients

The principle is for you to be able to use the feedback in discussion with an independent person, to facilitate reflection and generate an action plan for your own learning and implement the plan. Some MSF tools are available on Royal College and Faculty websites, so it is useful to explore these to assess if they meet your needs as an appraisee. We will briefly consider the following questionnaires:

1 The Doctors Interpersonal Skills Questionnaire (DISQ)
2 The Patient Enablement Instrument (PEI)
3 The Patient Satisfaction Questionnaire (PSQ)
4 The General Practice Assessment Questionnaire (GPAQ)

The Doctors Interpersonal Skills Questionnaire

The Doctors Interpersonal Skills Questionnaire (DISQ) was developed for use in primary care and has been used across the globe (Chisholm and Askham 2006). The DISQ was developed as a 16-item questionnaire with good psychometric properties, with intellectual property rights sitting within a private organization, the Client Focused Evaluations Program (CFEP). The original version has since been revised into a generic questionnaire called the Interpersonal Skills Questionnaire (ISQ), which has been used with other health professions. Both of the questionnaires gather patients' views on consultations with a focus on the humanistic aspects of the interaction. The scales within the questionnaire assess how communication skills are used to build rapport, provide empathy, convey respect, give good explanations, and elicit concerns effectively.

The Patient Enablement Instrument (PEI)

The Patient Enablement Instrument (PEI) is a six-item patient-reported outcome measure (PROM) developed for use in general practice (Howie et al. 1998). It is designed to measure the quality of appointments with GPs. The PEI is essentially a generic PROM and is not disease-specific. It is made up of a number of elements: duration of the appointment, higher patient satisfaction, positive doctor–patient relationship, and higher levels of perceived empathy from the doctor. This questionnaire has been widely used across the world (Mead et al. 2008). Patients rate the consultation along a 4-point scale, from much better to less good or not applicable in their ability to:

• Understand their illness
• Cope with life
• Keep healthy
• Cope with illness
• Be confident about their health
• Be more able to help themselves.

This is simple to use and can help identify areas of patient's unmet needs (PUNs) and therefore the doctor's educational needs (DENs) as discussed later in this chapter (Eve 2003).

The Patient Satisfaction Questionnaire (PSQ)

The original Patient Satisfaction Questionnaire was an 80-item questionnaire designed for use in general population studies to help design clinical services. The 18-item version (PSQ-18) was developed for use in primary care (Marshall and Hays 1994) and has been validated for use in a wide range of clinical settings. The items map to a number of key domains from the original version. These are:

1 Satisfaction with the doctor
2 Access to services
3 Appointments
4 Facilities
5 Nurses
6 Global satisfaction

The patients rate the doctor on a 7-point scale, from 1 = poor to 7 = outstanding. Examples of questions are:

Rate the doctor at:

Putting you at ease
Letting you tell your story.

(Marshall and Hays 1994)

The General Practice Assessment Questionnaire (GPAQ)

The General Practice Assessment Questionnaire (GPAQ) is a shortened version of the General Practice Assessment Survey (GPAS) and is used in general practice (Chisholm and Askham 2006). It measures communication, engagement, interpersonal skills, as well as access to primary care services in general. The process also gathers limited demographic data from each patient, which can be used to compare and benchmark results.

Summary of MSFs

The purpose of MSF is for the appraisee to obtain feedback from patients and or colleagues who they interact with during the course of their work. The role of the appraisee is to reflect on the feedback and it is vital to avoid being defensive. One may not agree with the content of some feedback but that is what the participants have said, so the appraisee needs to reflect and consider what action is needed.

Patient-Reported Outcome Measures (PROMs) and Patient-Reported Experience Measures (PREMS)

The introduction of the concept of PROMs and patient-reported experience measures (PREMs) occurred in NHS England in 2009 (Devlin and Appleby 2010). These concepts were heralded as a major shift to improve the processes leading to the remodeling of services to meet the needs of patients.

The introduction of PROMs reflected a growing recognition across health systems in the world that the patient's perspective is vital in helping to shape any initiatives that aim to improve the quality and effectiveness of health care. The aspiration was that PROMs would be a key driver for how health and social care are funded, commissioned, and delivered.

The focus on PROMs and PREMs was in large part facilitated by the emerging drive to apply the principles of quality improvement methodology and the recognition of the need to consider health care in a systems manner. It recognized that the patients' view of the impact and value of any heath care intervention was important. The question started to be asked (Gray 2011): what value for the patient is achieved by the use of this particular resource?

The increasing focus on the value the patient assigns to any intervention was also echoed by Don Berwick, past President and Chief Executive of the Institute for Healthcare Improvement:

> *The ultimate measure by which to judge the quality of a medical effort is whether it helps patients (and their families) as they see it. Anything done in health care that does not help a patient or family is, by definition, waste, whether or not the professions and their associations traditionally hallow it.*
>
> (Berwick 1997)

In the context of appraisal there is an opportunity to use PROMs and PREMs to enable the individual practitioner, and also the team they work in, to reflect, learn and change behavior.

There are simple tools available to gather data on an ongoing basis that can be used to improve services to individuals and groups, but also useful for individual doctors to use to generate learning.

In the field of mental health, one example of such a tool is DIALOG+ (Priebe et al. 2007). This is an app-based therapeutic intervention using a series of simple questions that the patient answers on a regular basis. The aim is to improve the communication between a health professional and the patient, and through that the outcomes of mental health care. It combines assessment, planning, intervention, and evaluation in one relatively simple process. Patients are asked to answer a series of 11 questions rating their satisfaction on a 7-point scale, where 1 is totally dissatisfied and 7 is totally satisfied. The questions are shown in Table 5.1.

Table 5.1 Questions used in DIALOG+.

1. How satisfied are you with your mental health?
2. How satisfied are you with your physical health?
3. How satisfied are you with your job situation?
4. How satisfied are you with your accommodation?
5. How satisfied are you with your leisure activities?
6. How satisfied are you with your relationship with your partner/family?
7. How satisfied are you with your friendships?
8. How satisfied are you with your personal safety?
9. How satisfied are you with your medication?
10. How satisfied are you with the practical help you receive?
11. How satisfied are you with your meetings with mental health professionals?

Source: Adapted from Priebe et al. (2007).

One of the principles of using data is not to re-invent the wheel. The aim is to use either data that are already gathered on a routine, automated basis or to use a simple tool. One of the advantages with DIALOG+ is that it is simple for patients to engage with and for staff to use. Patients use an app on a device to complete the scale in the meeting with their clinicians. The ratings are then used by the patient with the clinicians to focus on key areas that they are most concerned about. Each concern is then addressed in a systematic approach using four steps: understanding the problem; agreeing the best outcome; exploring options with the patient and what others can do to achieve the patient's desired outcome; and then agreeing actions.

This process can be used to identify individual and team learning needs mapped to the patient's unmet need, similar to the concept of PUNS (Eve 2003).

Peer-to-peer Support

Peer-to-peer support can be used to help reflection on potential areas for development, and for someone else who perhaps understands the clinical and wider context in which the appraisee is working to provide a sounding board. This approach includes Royal College (RC) CPD support groups. The purpose of these, in general, is to sign off the CPD the appraisee has undertaken and also to act as a forum for targeted CPD that all members of that group consider to be appropriate. This can take the form of learning using tools such as case-based discussion. Peer groups can be driven by RC processes which, although useful, are not now mandatory for appraisal and revalidation. It could be argued that the CPD points-gathering is a rather old-fashioned and educationally unsound process. Recording that you attended an online webinar or lecture without then reflecting is meaningless.

For example, on the Royal College of Psychiatrists (RCPsych) website it states:

CPD Submissions [part of the College website] lets you log your CPD activity and peer group membership and generate a RCPsych CPD certificate of good standing. If you're working in a non-training grade and have a GMC licence to practise, you'll need to evidence your CPD.

(Royal College of Psychiatrists 2021)

So with this example, "being in good standing" with one's College is not required for revalidation but rather engagement with appraisal over five cycles. Of course there may be other accreditations/skills that need you be to be in good standing with one's college. In Wales, as an example, this is one of the criteria required to fulfill the training requirements to be an Approved Clinician for the purposes of the Mental Health Act. So it is worthwhile checking with your specialty or college.

Mentoring/Coaching
Mentoring
Mentorship schemes in medicine are relatively common. Some Royal Colleges support and provide mentoring, and employers have focused on offering mentors particularly to newly appointed consultants. There are a range of definitions of mentoring, but a useful one offered by Megginson and Clutterbuck (1995) is as follows:

Help by one person to another in making significant transitions in knowledge, work or thinking.

(Megginson and Clutterbuck 1995, p. 5)

One of the main purposes of any mentoring relationship is to help the mentee to maximize their potential, both in terms of what they do on a day-to-day basis and in terms of career aspirations. In the context of appraisal and revalidation the mentee can use the discussions in this relationship to identify unmet learning need.

In general, there are two types of mentorship relationship, informal and formal. With the latter, it may be that within the organization you work, there is a scheme whereby individuals are identified as potential mentors and are trained and work to a certain set of rules. In more formal and systematic approaches there are typically rules of engagement that may involve the following:

1 The choice in regard to the frequency and type of communication is led by the mentee.
2 The agreed role of the mentor is to act as a sounding board. In particular the mentor does not advise or tell the mentee what to do.

3 The mentoring relationship is a two-way process based on mutual respect. There should be no hierarchy.

4 The relationship should be characterized as "a relationship between equals" (Hay 1999).

The length of the mentoring relationship can vary depending on the needs of the mentee. It is common, however, for the arrangement to be more long term.

As with all relationships one has to be aware that the mentor/mentee relationship can potentially become quite destructive. This has been described by David Clutterbuck (2004) as the "toxic mentor", characterized by:

1 The mentor regularly inappropriately bringing their issues and problems to the relationship.

2 The mentor follows their own alternative agenda that does meet the needs of the mentee.

3 If the mentee chooses not to follow the advice given, the mentor may take offense.

Coaching

There are different types of coaching including career, life, performance, and leadership coaching. In a mentoring relationship the mentor tends to be more experienced and the relationship is mutually beneficial. In coaching, the role for the coach is different and all types of coaching share the same themes including:

1 A partnership relationship

2 A goal-focused approach, not aimed at developing the person more broadly

3 A focus on the here and now and what the client wants to achieve

4 Understanding the client's perspective and also their current situation, their reality

5 Similar to mentoring, there needs to be a safe and confidential relationship

6 Maximizing an individual's personal and professional potential.

Coaching aims to enhance the individual's self-awareness, and in the context of appraisal this should help facilitate reflection.

There are many models that are used to structure task/goal orientated conversations such as the Association for Talent Development (ATD) COACH (ATD 2021) and the GROW model (Whitmore 2009). This latter model is explored in more detail in Chapter 4. A brief description of the four-step ATD COACH model is as follows.

Step 1 Current situation – the coach and the client come to a mutual understanding of the current situation. Understanding where a client is starting from is key in developing realistic objectives.

Step 2 Objectives – agree measurable end-goal objectives that are realistic and achievable.

Step 3 Alternatives – explore alternative options to achieve the objectives.

Step 4 Choices – the creation of a plan of action that includes milestones and, if needed, coaching follow-ups.

At the end of step 4, the client should have a clear path forward with measurable ways of progressing toward their objective. Through a coaching process, it is common to identify unmet learning needs, and this can be useful to reflect on and plan action.

The Johari Window

The Johari window (Luft and Ingham 1950) is a relatively simple tool to help explore one's perceived and true learning needs (see Figure 5.1). The purpose of the Johari window is to facilitate personal self-awareness, and it has been adapted for use in a wide range of settings. It is particularly useful in educational/training settings. In the context of the appraisal process it can be used to aid reflection. The tool is visually represented as four windows that facilitate personal self-awareness.

In the context of learning needs, panes 1 and 3 reflect the learner's awareness of their own learning needs, and as such represent the individual's perceived learning needs. In pane 1, the learning needs are also known by someone external, the trainer, supervisor or coach. However, in pane 3, these needs are known only by the learner.

Panes 2 and 4 reflect learning needs that the learner does not have insight to. In pane 2 the learning needs are unknown by the individual but known to others and in pane 4 neither the learner nor external person are aware of learning needs. Therefore, panes 2 and 4 represent the true learning needs.

	Learning needs known to learner	Learning needs unknown to learner
Learning needs known to tutor	1 Open	4 Blind
Learning needs unknown to tutor	3 Hidden	4 Unknown

Figure 5.1 The Johari window adapted for use in an educational setting. Source: Adapted from Luft and Ingham (1950).

This simple approach can be used in practice after, for example, a mentoring discussion or peer-to-peer group meeting, allowing the individual to reflect particularly upon their unknown learning needs.

Strengths, Weaknesses, Opportunities, Threats (SWOT) Analysis
SWOT (strengths, weaknesses, opportunities and threats) analysis is widely used in the business world to identify and analyze any factors, both internal and external, that can have an impact on the viability of a project, product, place or person. SWOT analysis can also be used by individuals as a tool for personal reflection and hence can be useful to support appraisal (The Open University 2017). Strengths and weaknesses relate to your own internal factors. The first step is to reflect on your strengths as evidenced by any feedback you have had via MSF or any other source over the last appraisal cycle. The next step is to reflect on any opportunities in this context from learning that you can think of, and then consider any threats, highlight constraints or challenges you think you may encounter (see Table 5.2). This could include access to the right training or funding (see challenges later in this chapter). These represent the external factors at play.

With this process the opportunities lead on to an action plan for learning.

Patient's Unmet Needs (PUNs) and Doctor's Educational Needs (DENs)
One approach to identifying one's learning needs is to begin with the question of the patient's unmet needs (PUNs) (Eve 2003). This is an alternative way of recording the patient experience, similar to PROMs and PREMs discussed above. Although this simple process was first described in General Practice, it is applicable in any clinical setting. The idea is to spot the PUN, then define the learning that you need to meet the PUN. This approach is supported by the concept that as doctors we are adult learners, and as such any new learning builds on one's personal experience, adds to prior learning, and leads to the spiral of recognizing the need for further learning. The focus with PUNs is for the learning to be directly linked to improving patient care.

Table 5.2 Example of a simple SWOT analysis.

Strengths	Weaknesses
I can do . . . very well	I am not so good at doing . . .
Opportunities	**Threats**
I am aware that colleagues in a nearby cluster/hospital provide opportunity to observe . . .	Getting time away from the practice will be a challenge. I will need support of my colleagues.

The starting point is the patient's real needs and not their stated wants. This is a process that occurs at every clinical interaction. With any unmet patient need, this should drive the doctor's learning to meet those needs. You may enjoy learning about childhood asthma. Using this model that is your wants, but if you are already competent in this area and the process is telling you that patients with depression as a group have unmet needs, then this should dictate your learning, for the benefit of patients and not your own benefit (Figure 5.2).

How do you do this in practice? Eve was in GP and suggested that the practice team undertake a week-long exercise where each clinician asks themselves the question: was I equipped to meet this patient's needs?

Once identifying a PUN, Eve suggests categorizing them into the following:
- Clinical knowledge
- Non-clinical
- Skill or attitude.

This approach can the facilitate identifying how you can access learning to meet the needs.

Individual vs Team Learning Needs

It is important to recognize that no single doctor can meet all of the health care needs of every single patient. This then brings into sharp focus the importance of team working, interprofessional learning and delegation. The importance of interprofessional education and the positive impact on patient experience and outcomes have been extensively reported (Strasser et al. 2008; Janson et al. 2009). We will briefly consider the area of delegation, for completeness.

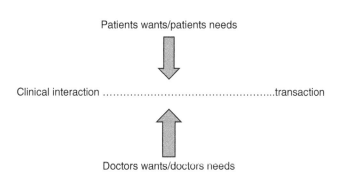

Patients wants/patients needs

Clinical interaction ....transaction

Doctors wants/doctors needs

Figure 5.2 Patient wants and needs versus doctor wants and needs. Source: Adapted from Eve (2003).

Delegation

The GMC have produced very useful guidance (GMC 2020b), as have all other regulators in heath, on your role and responsibilities in a delegation scenario. They also usefully provide clarity between delegation and referral.

From the GMC recent guidance, the following are key elements that need consideration:

Delegation involves asking a colleague to provide care or treatment on your behalf.

When delegating care, you must be satisfied that the person to whom you delegate has the knowledge, skills and experience to provide the relevant care or treatment; or that the person will be adequately supervised. If you are delegating to a person who is not registered with a statutory regulatory body, voluntary registration can provide some assurance that practitioners have met defined standards of competence and adhere to agreed standards for their professional skills and behaviour. When you delegate care you are still responsible for the overall management of the patient.

(GMC 2020b)

In regard to referral, the GMC clarification states:

Referral is when you arrange for another practitioner to provide a service that falls outside your professional competence. Usually you will refer to another doctor or healthcare professional registered with a statutory regulatory body. Where this is not the case, you must be satisfied that systems are in place to assure the safety and quality of care provided – for example, the services have been commissioned through an NHS commissioning process or the practitioner is on a register accredited by the Professional Standards Authority.

You must also follow our guidance in paragraph 26–33 of Sharing information for direct care. General Medical Council (2017) Confidentiality: good practice in handling patient information, London, GMC.

(GMC 2020b)

The process of delegating requires specific skills and this is an area that you may want to consider as a learning need.

National Audits

Some RCs and related organizations undertake audits that provide benchmarked normative data, including outcomes that can be useful in helping to generate PDPs. One example is the National Emergency Laparotomy Audit

(NELA). This is an annual UK audit of outcomes for emergency laparotomies and is carried out by the National Institute of Academic Anaesthesia's Health Service Research Centre, on behalf of the Royal College of Anaesthetists.

It is stated on the NELA website:

> *NELA aims to enable the improvement of the quality of care for patients undergoing emergency laparotomy, through the provision of high quality comparative data from all providers of emergency laparotomy.*
>
> *NELA is being carried out. . . with surgical and other key stakeholders.*
>
> *Please keep in mind that NELA is on ongoing audit and that the data collection process continues as usual.*
>
> (NELA 2021)

NELA provides data on a number of parameters down to hospital-level performance indicators benchmarked to agreed service standards. NELA covers a wide range of criteria and include the following as examples:

- Computed tomography reported before surgery by a consultant radiologist
- Consultant surgeon present in theater when risk of death ≥25%
- Admitted to critical care post-op when risk of death ≥10%
- Risk-adjusted mortality within 30 days of surgery.

The overview provides:

- Total number of patients included
- Overall hospital performance
- Average performance across all hospitals
- RAG rating (red–amber–green) of overall performance.

Another UK-wide audit is the National Cancer Diagnosis Audit (NCDA) led by Cancer Research UK (2021). This audit records primary and secondary care data relating to patients diagnosed with cancer. The data is shared with the participants with the aim of increasing understanding of the cancer pathways and highlighting what is working well and what areas require improvement.

The audit drills down to data such as:

> The time from the patient first presenting to diagnosis
> Symptoms on assessment
> Patient characteristics
> The use of investigations in primary care prior to referral
> What the referral pathways for patients with cancer are and how they compare with those recorded by the cancer registry.

The NCDA data is analyzed centrally for free and each GP practice receives a confidential, tailored feedback report.

All NHS employers, commissioners and those in the private sector will collect a wide range of data. These data can vary from process data such as the number of referrals into outpatients, number of patients seen once, and number referred onto other services. There is likely to be outcome data, depending on your specialty, of morbidity or mortality. It is useful to consider these data to trigger reflection on learning needs.

Clinical Governance Processes
Following a number of major failures in standards of care, and in particular the Bristol Royal Infirmary scandal (see Chapter 3 for more details), the UK government along with other stakeholders introduced the concept of clinical governance in 1999. This has been defined as:

> . . . *a framework through which UK National Health Service (NHS) organisations and their staff are accountable for continuously improving the quality of patient care. NHS staff need to ensure that the appropriate systems and processes are in place to monitor clinical practice and safeguard high quality of care. Clinical governance is central to the UK Government's agenda to ensure that quality of care becomes a key driver in the development of health services.*

> (Department for International Development 2001)

Clinical governance is based upon seven underlying principles or pillars, and these can be remembered by using the mnemonic "PIRATES". The seven principles are:

> Patient and public involvement
> It is widely accepted that feedback from patients and the public in general is central to any changes to service delivery. The involvement of the public and patients can be achieved by gathering feedback from them in regards to many aspects of their care via surveys and informal and formal consultative meetings.
> Information and IT
> The appropriate use of accurate data is a key component in the process of improving the quality of clinical services. It is important to use information technology (IT) to monitor service delivery and measure quality outcomes. Any use of IT must ensure patient confidentiality at all times.
> Risk management
> Risk management is defined as a systematic and cyclic process to achieve the following:
> > Identify risk

Assess the risks for likelihood and potential severity
Eliminate the risks that can be eliminated
Reduce the effect of those risks that cannot be eliminated
Acknowledge formally those risks that can be accepted
Monitor risk
Review level of risks
Any risk management framework should enable any significant events to be learned from and foster a blame-free culture in which risks and mistakes may be reported without fear of reprisals.

Audit
A comprehensive and multi-professional audit process is central for ensuring that the quality of services meet or exceed agreed standards. Through this process any shortfalls in the standard of care are addressed and are then subject to further cycles of audit to ensure that any improvements are maintained.

Training and education
A central element to clinical governance is the need to have an ongoing program of training and education for all staff to continue to perform their roles at the top of their competency ceiling. In addition, top-up training allows staff to enhance their skills in line with an ever-changing and evolving clinical practice setting. So the identification of learning needs for individuals and clinical teams can be used in appraisal reflections to help generate learning needs.

Effectiveness in clinical care
Effectiveness in providing clinical care requires delivery units to implement and adhere to national standards and guidelines. Central to achieving this is to take an evidence-based approach to patient care and conducting research that adds to existing evidence in order to enhance future standards of patient care.

Staff management
This concerns the need in clinical governance for effective staff recruitment and management, including performance monitoring and improvement and, where necessary, team and morale-building, motivation and the establishment of a sound working environment.

In any clinical practice significant events will occur and the pillars of clinical governance should facilitate learning at an individual, team, departmental and organizational level. Analysis of significant events can be an invaluable tool to help identify individual and team learning needs. Significant events can include a wide variety of events both good and bad, including the following:

- Letter of complaint
- Staff issues

- Compliments from patients/relatives
- Delay in cancer diagnosis
- Unexpected death

Significant event analysis (SEA) has been defined by Gillam and Siriwardena (2013) as:

> the process by which individual cases, in which there has been a signifi-
> cant occurrence (not necessarily involving an undesirable outcome for
> the patient), are analysed in a systematic and detailed way to ascertain
> what can be learnt about the overall quality of care and to indicate
> changes that might lead to future improvements.
>
> (Gillam and Siriwardena 2013, p. 126)

The stated aims of SEA are:

1 To use lessons learnt to improve quality of care
2 To identify good practice as well as not so good practice
3 To foster a no-blame and open and honest culture
4 To be a tool to help identify CPD.

Datix is the widely used reporting system in the NHS for recording clinical incidents or "near misses." It allows for the sharing of the details of incidents, enabling weaknesses in the system to be identified, customs and practices to be changed, and staff to be retrained where necessary. Datix allows incidents to be reported in real-time, reducing the delays experienced with paper systems. The system was established in 1986 by Brian Capstick, founder of a law firm specializing in defending NHS organizations against clinical negligence claims.

Know Yourself – Know your Learning Styles

To maximize your time, it is useful to be aware of how you learn. This is called your preferred learning style. We all naturally tend to use certain ways to learn. This is the way you naturally learn and frequently we may be unaware of the ways in which we can maximize our learning. There are various models, but a useful one is the "Learning Styles" approach (Honey and Mumford 1986). They describe four different learning styles:

1 Activists
2 Reflectors
3 Theorists
4 Pragmatists

They developed a simple Learning Styles Questionnaire (Honey and Mumford 2000) consisting of 80 questions. You are able to score your answer to get a total score on each of the four main learning styles. This can be useful to help individuals to identify the most appropriate type of learning experience.

Activists

Those whose learning style is characterized by the activist tend to be flexible in approach, open-minded, and enjoy being exposed to new experiences. They learn best by being thrown in at the deep end and enjoy being front and center, in the limelight. There is a tendency for them to thrive on new challenges, but there is a risk that they get bored with implementation and longer-term consolidation.

Reflectors

Those individuals with a reflective learning style tend to observe, collect data/information, and then reflect on all of that thoroughly before coming to any conclusion. The thorough collection and analysis of data about experiences and events is very important and they will tend not to jump to conclusions. They require time to make decisions, and prefer to be more in the background, taking a back seat. Their philosophy is to be cautious and they learn least well if forced into situations without prior notice or planning.

Theorists

Theorists learn best in situations where the learning is presented in the context of, or underpinned by, a theoretical model or concept. Similar to the reflectors, they require time to consider information and to assimilate it, and they do this in a linear, step-by-step logical way. They will tend to need to be able to question and probe theories or model/assumptions and enjoy analyzing very complex concepts. They tend to have a disciplined and logical approach. They will tend to learn less well in situations where emotions and feelings are front and center, or are the focus.

Pragmatists

Those with a preferred learning style of the pragmatist are keen on trying out ideas, theories and techniques to see if they work in practice. The learning is optimized if they can see the direct link with what they do on a day-to-day basis, that is, they can see the practical application of the learning. They enjoy the immediacy of rehearsing newly learnt practical skills in, for example, a simulated environment, and getting immediate direct feedback from the coach/trainer/teacher. They tend to have a very business-like approach and prefer clear action plans with realistic objectives.

As with most concepts, there are overlaps between the four styles, and most individuals will have perhaps two styles that characterize their dominant learning. The most common combinations with this model are:

• First – Reflector/theorist
• Second – Theorist/pragmatist

- Third – Reflector/pragmatist
- Fourth – Activist/pragmatist

Another model of learning styles to mention briefly is the VARK model (Fleming 2017). This is an inventory designed to help students learn more about their individual learning preferences. According to the VARK model, learners are identified by whether they have a preference for:

- **V**isual learning (pictures, movies, diagrams)
- **A**uditory learning (music, discussion, lectures)
- **R**eading and writing (making lists, reading textbooks, taking notes)
- **K**inesthetic learning (movement, experiments, hands-on activities)

Reflection

Reflective Cycles and Action Plans

The ability to produce an effective reflection begins with having insight, and understanding the need to reflect. It is from here that we are able to understand where we are with our current areas of knowledge and areas for improvement. Once we have insight to this, we are then able to use various techniques to identify our specific learning needs. It is also important to recognize that the process of reflecting is a skill that can be learned and refined. In this context it is useful to explore some of the basic theory and models underpinning adult learning.

All adults use reflection to learn (Knowles 1980). The process of reflection is a basic tool used by humans to make sense of complex or ambiguous situations and learn from these experiences. There are a range of definitions of reflection and a useful one is (Moon 1999, p. 37):

> . . .*a form of mental processing – like a form of thinking – that we may use to fulfil a purpose or to achieve some anticipated outcome . . . reflection is applied to relatively complicated, ill-structured ideas for which there is not an obvious solution.*

The work of Schon (1983) highlighted the important concept of the reflective practitioner and described two types of reflection. The first is our reflections, our thinking at the time of the event or incident. This is called *reflection-in-action*. Sometime after the event we reflect more, *reflection-on-action*. Both of these processes facilitate learning from one experience being incorporated into future *knowing-in-action*.

Kolb (1984) described a four-stage model of reflective practice based on experiential learning that is applicable for learning in clinical practice. This is shown in Figure 5.3.

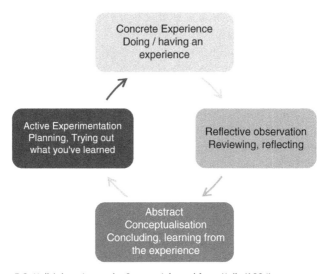

Figure 5.3 Kolb's learning cycle. Source: Adapted from Kolb (1984).

With Kolb's cycle the experience of an event in itself is not enough to promote learning. The individual must reflect and, in doing so, make links between theory and action in order to truly promote learning. In order to close the "learning gap" between the learner's current performance and their expected level, there is a need for an action plan. The SMART approach is a widely used method for generating well-structured and meaningful action plans that can be used irrespective of the reflective model that is used.

- Specific: learning outcomes need to be clearly stated in simple language.
- Measurable: must be able to measure the outcome so that the learner and others can have confidence it has been achieved.
- Achievable: all objectives must be realistic and achievable within the time-frame and with the resources available.
- Relevant: all learning objectives must be personally relevant to the learner, otherwise barriers to learning will develop.
- Timely: each objective must be time-bound with specific deadlines, and if needed, milestones can help assessment of progress.

Models of Reflection

There are a number of models of reflection. A useful resource produced by the Academy of Medical Royal Colleges (AoMRC) and the Conference of Postgraduate Medical Deans (COPMeD) (AoMRC and COPMeD 2018) gives examples of different models of reflection, including Rolfe et al. (2001) and the Gibbs Reflective Cycle (Gibbs 1988). Most doctors find that a certain model is a best fit for them. We will briefly describe these two models, along with the Dewey reflective spiral (Dewey 1938).

Rolfe and Colleagues

One advantage with the model described by Rolfe et al. (2001) is that it is simple and straightforward. This model can be distilled down to three "what" questions: *What? So what? Now what?*

The first "what" question is really an exploration of what happened and reflections on the impact of this on others and yourself.

What. . .
> Happened?
> Was my role in what happened?
> Was I trying to achieve?
> Did I do to try and achieve this?
> Were the responses of other people involved?
> Were the consequences?

The next "so what" question is about reflecting on why the event was important and exploring whether you could have handled things in any other ways.

So what. . .
> Were my thought processes throughout the 'event'?
> Other approaches might I have used?
> Else could be done to produce a better outcome?
> Have I learned because of this situation?
> Does this tell me about myself and my relationships with those involved?

The next "now what" question is about pulling together all aspects of the event or situation and thinking about what you could do differently in the future, if faced with a similar set of circumstances. Now what. . .
> Do I need to do to improve my performance?
> Have I learned about myself?
> Have I learned about others?
> Will I do differently in the future?

Gibbs Reflective Cycle

Another reflective model is that of Gibbs (1988), which differs from Rolf and colleagues with the addition of the key stage of reflecting on how you felt, your emotional state at the time of the event. This is best described graphically as in Figure 5.4.

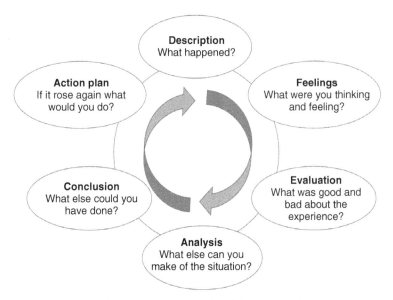

Figure 5.4 Gibbs Reflective Cycle. Source: Adapted from Gibbs (1988).

The stages of Gibbs are:

1 The description
   The first step is to describe the event or situation.

2 Feelings
   You then reflect on your emotional state and associated thinking at the time of the event. A question to ask yourself is: how did my emotions affect my thinking and subsequent behavior?

3 Evaluation
   At this point reflect on how you handled the situation. What were the good aspects and what would you consider doing differently?

4 Conclusion
   This is really a summary stage when you consider any other aspects and in particular any alternative options that you would use if faced with a similar set of circumstances in the future. Also, what did you learn from this event that you could transfer to other situations?

5 Action plan
   At this stage you identify any action you need to take. This could include training or upskilling. The key point is for you to be clear what you will do to ensure that any learning is embedded and determines your behavior in the future.

One of the advantages with the Gibbs cycle is that it provides a more systematic approach than that of Rolfe and colleagues. On the other hand the emphasis on description, it could be argued, produces a more superficial reflection.

Dewey's Reflective Spiral

Of course, in real-life medicine, there is an argument that the above models are too simplistic and perhaps unidimensional (Miettinen 2000).

The concept of experiential adult learning as a learning spiral founded on reflective thought and then action had been described by Dewey (1938) before Kolb's work. A key element in Dewey's theory was the need for learners to engage directly with their environment, the experiential aspect of learning. In this way individuals build on learning experiences and progress.

It could be argued that this developmental spiral fits better into the role of appraisal in an individual's professional progression. The whole concept of training in medicine and professional development is one of accumulating experience, knowledge and the skills to undertake practical procedures. Self-awareness of limitations and asking for help, where appropriate, are essential components of safe medical practice. The appraisal discussion is an ideal opportunity to demonstrate development and to discuss current limitations and future aspirations.

Based on Dewey's model of reflection, thinking, and then action, the appraisal spiral is shown in Figure 5.5 (Miettinen 2000). So in the context of appraisal your reflective thinking fuels the spiral and leads to a continuous cycle of reflection and learning.

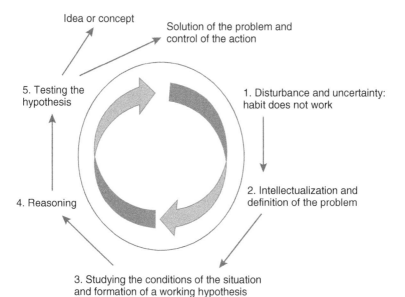

Figure 5.5 Dewey's reflective spiral. Source: Adapted from Miettinen (2000).

How you present your reflections will depend on where you work in the UK and on your personal preferences. All of the above models are acceptable processes to follow to gain the most from your appraisal.

Discuss

When preparing for your appraisal it is useful to consider what you want to focus on during the discussion. As mentioned above, it is not the quantity of entries that is important, it is the quality and how meaningful they are to you and the potential impact any learning might have on improving the quality of care to patients.

If you have used a mentor or coach to generate some of the reflections, then discussing the event and your reflections with them before the appraisal meeting may help you to refine your thinking.

And perhaps if you are a member of a CPD group it might be useful to use those colleagues to reflect on the key issues. This peer-to-peer support is very useful to help you to sense-check the areas you feel you want to focus on.

It is important to remember that the aim of appraisal is for you to get the most out of the discussion. It is not about getting it done, or getting it over with.

Action

A key question is: what has happened/changed as a result of your learning? Has there been a measurable improvement in the quality of patient care? If so, what evidence do you have for that? One example could be an audit showing improved adherence to anti-hypertensive medication with resultant increased percentage of patients with blood pressure measurements within an acceptable range, hence reducing risk of morbidity (the net outcome being a reduced risk of cerebrovascular accidents).

Challenges you may Face in the Process

There are many challenges to succeeding at the current appraisal and revalidation process. At a practical level, more and more doctors are opting for portfolio careers whereby some of the working week is not engaged in face-to-face with patients. How do you reflect on these so-called non-clinical roles and generate learning needs? Yet you will need to do this to be able to be in a position to maintain your license to practice in the clinical setting. We will briefly explore a number of common challenges including:

1 Finding the appropriate learning
2 Time available
3 Funding/support from the employer
4 Other challenges

Finding the Appropriate Learning

So you have reflected, discussed and agreed with the appraiser that there is a knowledge gap in a certain area. How do you go about sourcing the most appropriate learning? This is a balance of sourcing learning that will meet your learning needs. You can ask colleagues, check with your Royal College or Faculty, and check with your local employer or university.

One of the challenges with accessing the most appropriate learning is that not all delivering organizations are clear about the learning outcomes their activity is geared toward. Most conferences will only provide general aims of the sessions, and it can be difficult to see where and in what session you will get what you are looking for.

One action is to contact the organizers and explain your specific needs and ask them for their learning objectives. Of course, there may not be one single source that can help you to achieve your needs. You may need to attend/experience a number of events.

Time

Your needs may be best met by spending time within another department to observe new procedures for example. But even a day away from your clinical work may be a challenge. Within busy jobs it may be a challenge finding the time to be released for any CPD. It is all too easy to get stuck on the treadmill of clinical or other medical work and not have the headspace. This is in part why appraisal and revalidation were introduced. If you have used a recognized process to identify learning needs that will, with a level of evidence, lead to an improvement in patient outcomes or experience, it becomes more difficult for your employer not to allow the time for you to undertake that CPD. To aid engagement with your employer, it is useful to have discussions with your line manager to check whether what you feel is a key objective for you chimes with the employer's strategy

A skill to have and enhance is that of influencing. This is not only useful in the situation of negotiating time away from your own clinical practice for learning, but a useful generic skill. We use these influencing skills on others on a day-to-day basis.

Influencing is when we change someone's views, beliefs and/or decisions to produce a positive effect. The skills required include the following:

Active listening and asking probing questions
Building rapport
Building trust and credibility
Finding things in common to share – developing affinity
Being clear about your aim and having a plan
Being clear who your target group is – who is it that makes the decision you need?
Developing the skill of being assertive.

There are many useful resources on how to enhance your influencing skills (Gillen 1995).

Funding/Support from Employer

There may be a difference between what you want and what the patients and, to some extent, your employer needs or wants. What do you do if all agree that your skills would be enhanced and, as a result, patient outcomes would be improved if you were funded and supported to undertake XXX, but it doesn't happen. This can be extremely frustrating and can lead to a high level of dissatisfaction and disengagement with the process of appraisal.

Other Challenges

Life and worldwide events do and will continue to shape heath care and how all of us in that system work and learn. In 2020 the outbreak of the COVID-19 infection and the subsequent pandemic has had far-reaching and catastrophic consequences. In health care systems across the world, doctors are adjusting how they operate on a daily basis.

Routine work was generally frozen and then unfrozen. All of these changes have put unprecedented pressure on a normally pressurized system. This has been recognized by the GMC (GMC 2020c) who agreed that any doctor who was scheduled to revalidate between March 2020 and March 2021 would have their revalidation date moved on by 12 months.

One significant development has been the acceleration of the use of video consultations (VCs) in both GP and secondary care. This has been a necessity as a result of the pandemic, but there had already been increasing use of this method of consultation pre-COVID, particularly for patients with chronic conditions (Ignatowicz et al. 2019).

There have been mixed views about the use of technology in this way. One GP stated that the restrictions and resultant use of VCs have led her to practice substandard, second-best medicine (Salisbury 2020). Although these approaches are challenges, they are also opportunities to reflect and identify learning needs in the use of technology.

Chapter Summary

In this chapter we have set out the processes that, if followed, will help you prepare and experience a meaningful appraisal. We have described the key principles as set out by the GMC. We have provided examples of a wide range of tools and approaches that can be used to help identify learning needs. These included examples of MSF tools, peer-to-peer support, mentoring/coaching, and clinical governance processes. In addition, we have explored learning styles as a means to maximize one's learning.

A number of models of reflection are described including Gibbs and Kolb's learning cycles and others that can be useful in a practical way within a clinical setting. We also reflect on some challenges that any doctor may face, including lack of funding and pressures on time to be able to access learning.

References

Academy of Medical Royal Colleges and Conference of Postgraduate Medical Deans (2018). *Academy and COPMeD Reflective Practice Toolkit.* https://www.copmed.org.uk/images/docs/reflective_practice/Reflective_Practice_Toolkit.pdf (accessed 12 May 2021).

Association for Talent Development (2021). *ATD COACH. What is Executive Coaching?* https://www.td.org/talent-development-glossary-terms/what-is-executive-coaching (accessed 15 May 2021).

Berwick, D.M. (1997). Medical associations: guilds or leaders? *British Medical Journal* **314** (7094): 1564–1565. https://doi.org/10.1136/bmj.314.7094.1564.

Cancer Research UK (2021). *National Cancer Diagnosis Audit. Audit to improve care.* Cancer Research UK. https://www.cancerresearchuk.org/health-professional/diagnosis/national-cancer-diagnosis-audit/audit-to-improve-care (accessed 10 May 2021).

Chisholm, A. and Askham, J. (2006). *What Do you Think of your Doctor?* Oxford: Picker Institute Europe.

Clutterbuck, D. (2004). *Everyone Needs a Mentor.* UK: CIPD.

Department for International Development (2001). *Clinical Governance in the UK NHS.* London: Department for International Development Health Systems Resource Centre. https://assets.publishing.service.gov.uk/media/57a08d59ed915d622c001935/Clinical-governance-in-the-UK-NHS.pdf (accessed 10 May 2021).

Devlin, N. J. and Appleby, J. (2010). *Getting the most out of PROMs. Putting health outcomes at the heart of NHS decision-making.* London: The King's Fund.

Dewey, J. (1938). *Logic. The Theory of Inquiry. The Later Works of John Dewey,* vol. **12** (ed. J.A. Boyston). Carbondale & Edwardsville: Southern Illinois University Press.

Eve, R. (2003). *PUNs and DENs. Discovering learning needs in general practice.* CRC Press.

Fleming, N. (2017). The VARK modalities. http://vark-learn.com/introduction-to-vark/the-vark-modalities (accessed 16 May 2021).

General Medical Council (2020a). *Guidance on Supporting Information for Appraisal and Revalidation*. London: General Medical Council.

General Medical Council (2020b). *Delegation and referral*. London: General Medical Council. https://www.gmc-uk.org/ethical-guidance/ethical-guidance-for-doctors/delegation-and-referral (accessed 10 May 2021).

General Medical Council (2020c). Changes to revalidation in response to COVID. http://gmc-uk.org (accessed 1 February 2021).

General Medical Council (2021a). Resources for collecting feedback. https://www.gmc-uk.org/registration-and-licensing/managing-your-registration/revalidation/revalidation-resources (accessed 16 May 2021).

General Medical Council (2021b). Our case studies on seeking patient feedback. https://www.gmc-uk.org/registration-and-licensing/managing-your-registration/revalidation/revalidation-resources#revalidation-patient-case-studies (accessed 16 May 2021).

Gibbs, G. (1988). *Learning by Doing. A Guide to Teaching and Learning Methods*. Oxford: Oxford Polytechnic.

Gillam, S. and Siriwardena, A.N. (2013). Frameworks for improvement: clinical audit, the plan-do-study-act cycle and significant event audit. *Quality in Primary Care* 21: 123–130.

Gillen, T. (1995). *Positive Influencing Skills (Developing Skills)*. Chartered Institute of Personnel and Development.

Gray, J.A.M. (2011). *How to Build Healthcare Systems*. Offox Press for Better Value Healthcare Ltd.

Hay, J. (1999). *Transformational Mentoring – Creating Developmental Alliances for Changing Organizational Cultures*. Watford: Sherwood Publishing.

Honey, P. and Mumford, A. (1986). *Using your Learning Styles*. Maidenhead: Peter Honey Publications Ltd.

Honey, P. and Mumford, A. (2000). *The Learning Styles Helper's Guide*. Maidenhead: Peter Honey Publications Ltd.

Howie, J.G.R., Heaney, D., Maxwell, M. et al. (1998). A comparison of the patient enablement instrument (PEI) against two established satisfaction scales as an outcome measure of primary care consultations. *Family Practice* 15: 165–171.

Ignatowicz, A., Atherton, H., Bernstein, C.J. et al. (2019). Internet videoconferencing for patient–clinician consultations in long-term conditions: a review of reviews and applications in line with guidelines and recommendations. *Digit Health* 5:2055207619845831. doi:https://doi.org/10.1177/2055207619845831. pmid:31069105.

Janson, S.L., Cooke, M., McGrath, K.W. et al. (2009). Improving chronic care of Type 2 diabetes using teams of interprofessional learners. *Academic Medicine* 84: 1540–1548.

Knowles, M.S. (1980). *The Modern Practice of Adult Education: From Pedagogy to Andragogy*, 2e. New York: Cambridge Books.

Knowles, M.S., Swanson, R., and Holton, E. (2011). *The Adult Learner: The Definitive Classic in Adult Education and Human Resource Development*, 7e. Amsterdam: Elsevier.

Kolb, D.A. (1984). *Experiential Learning Experience as a Source of Learning and Development*. New Jersey: Prentice Hall.

Laxdal, O. (1982). Needs assessment in continuing medical education: a practical guide. *Journal of Medical Education* **57**: 827–834.

Lockyer, J. (1998). Needs assessment: lesson learned. *Journal of Continuing Education in the Health Professions* **18**: 190–192.

Luft, J. and Ingham, H. (1950). *The Johari window, a graphic model of interpersonal awareness*. In: *Proceedings of the Western Training Laboratory in Group Development*. Los Angeles: UCLA.

Marshall, G.N. and Hays, R.D. (1994). *The Patient Satisfaction Questionnaire Short Form (PSQ-18)*. Santa Monica, CA: RAND.

Mead, N., Bower, P., and Roland, M. (2008). Factors associated with enablement in general practice: cross-sectional study using routinely-collected data. *British Journal of General Practice* **58**: 346–352.

Medical Appraisal Scotland (2021). Welcome to Medical Appraisal Scotland (home of SOAR). https://www.appraisal.nes.scot.nhs.uk/ (accessed 16 May 2021).

Megginson, D. and Clutterbuck, D. (1995). *Mentoring in Action*. London: Kogan Page.

Miettinen, R. (2000). The concept of experiential learning and John Dewey's theory of reflective thought and action. *International Journal of Lifelong Education* **19** (1): 54–72. https://doi.org/10.1080/026013700293458.

Moon, J.A. (1999). *Learning Journals: A Handbook for Academics, Students and Professional Development*. London: Kogan Page.

National Emergency Laparotomy Audit (2021). Welcome to the National Emergency Laparotomy Audit (NELA). https://www.nela.org.uk (accessed 10 May 2021).

Priebe, S., McCabe, R., Bullenkamp, J. et al. (2007). Structured patient–clinician communication and 1-year outcome in community mental healthcare. *British Journal of Psychiatry* **191**: 420–426.

Rolfe, G., Freshwater, D., and Jasper, M. (2001). *Critical Reflection for Nursing and the Helping Professions: A User's Guide*. Basingstoke: Palgrave Macmillan.

Royal College of Psychiatrists (2021). Submitting your CPD. https://www.rcpsych.ac.uk/members/submitting-your-cpd (accessed 10 May 2021).

Salisbury, H. (2020). Teleconsultations for all. *British Medical Journal* **370**: m3211.

Sargeant, J., Armson, H., Chesluk, B. et al. (2010). The processes and dimensions on informed self-assessment: a conceptual model. *Academic Medicine* **85** (7): 1212–1220.

Schon, D.A. (1983). *The Reflective Practitioner: How Professionals Think in Action*. New York: Basic Books.

Strasser, D.C., Falconer, J.A., Stevens, A.B. et al. (2008). Team training and stroke rehabilitation outcomes: a cluster randomized trial. *Archives of Physical Medicine Rehabilitation* **89**: 10–15.

The Open University (2017). Business communication: writing a SWOT analysis. OpenLearn. The Open University. https://www.open.edu/openlearn/money-business/business-communication-writing-swot-analysis/content-section-1# (accessed 16 May 2021).

Whitmore, J. (2009). *Coaching for Performance*, 4e. London: Nicholas Brealey.

Chapter 6 **Examples of Reflections Across All GMC Domains**

Introduction

A key role of the appraisee is to identify and gather supporting information (SI), reflect on it, and generate a plan. A frequent challenge is the task of how to record the reflections into the process in a meaningful way. Across the UK there are many different systems and formats that are in use. However, the principles of medical revalidation are the same across the UK and are driven by the details in the previous two chapters.

In this chapter we will provide a range of examples of reflective entries. These are not exhaustive, and the aim is to give those who struggle with reflective writing a template for their own reflections and learning.

It can be a challenge to decide what to include in the SI. A key rule is quality above quantity. A useful question to ask is: what impact has this experience had on my clinical practice? It is more meaningful for the appraisee to focus on events that potentially can lead to more impact on clinical practice. The events that trigger reflections don't necessarily need to be a continuing professional development event or a national or international conference. Sometimes the most impactful experiences can be a conversation with a colleague or a patient that triggers thinking (reflecting), then taking steps to learn, and then putting that new learning into practice. This is the essence of Dewey's developmental spiral as discussed in Chapter 5 (Dewey 1938).

The Domains Revisited

The General Medical Council (GMC) have articulated four domains, overarching themes to which the appraisee has to map their SI (GMC 2020). Within each

How to Succeed at Revalidation, First Edition. Peter Donnelly and Katie Webb.
© 2022 John Wiley & Sons Ltd. Published 2022 by John Wiley & Sons Ltd.

of these there are attributes, and within each of these a set of principles and values.

These can appear somewhat daunting when faced with appraisal for the first time. Whatever the clinical area or specialty, there will be numerous events, interactions with patients, feedback formal and informal that will in the normal course of events lead to reflection and subsequently change in the appraisee's individual practice, or influence the practice of the wider clinical team, all for the benefit of patients. The ideal is that with reflective entries one can show how the learning changed day-to-day clinical practice for the benefit of patients. In such a complex system as the NHS. it can be a challenge to quantify these changes. However, one can give examples of patient interactions where, based on prior leaning, the intervention was revised, or that there was a feeling of more confidence in decision-making, and/or the patient experience or outcome improved.

The GMC Domains

The GMC domains as stated in GMP are (GMC 2020):
Domain 1: Skills, knowledge and performance
Domain 2: Safety and quality
Domain 3: Communication, partnership and teams
Domain 4: Maintaining trust
A lot of events and interactions will map to a number of domains, and most experiences are complex. There are six types of SI that must be collected. They are:

> **Continuing professional development**
> **Quality improvement activity**
> **Significant events or serious incidents**
> **Feedback from patients**
> **Feedback from colleagues**
> **Compliments and complaints**

Tables 6.1–6.4 contain summaries of the attributes, example of principles and values in each of the Domains (GMC 2020). These are adapted from GMC *Good Medical Practice* (GMC 2020), and in the third column we provide brief examples of potential content.

Table 6.1 Domain 1: Knowledge, skills and performance.

Attributes	Examples of principles and values	Examples of content that could be used
1.1 Develop and maintain your professional performance	Keep up to date with and follow the law, GMC guidance and other regulations relevant to your work	Reflecting on gaining consent from a patient with dementia–informed consent (Chan etal. 2017).
	Keep professional knowledge and skills up to date	Reflecting on a complex case of asthma presenting to you out of hours.
	Participate in activities that maintain and develop your competence and performance	Reflecting on a one-day update on managing complex asthma and how it has changed your practice and that of others you supervise.
	Take steps to monitor and improve the quality of your work	Reflecting on the national/local prescribing audit and how it has changed your prescribing.
1.2 Apply knowledge and experience to practice	Recognize and work within the limits of your competence	As a GP, reflecting on your lack of confidence in managing patients with psychosis and the multiple array of antipsychotics now used for mood disorders.
	If teacher/trainer, apply the skills, attitudes and practice of a competent teacher/trainer	Reflecting on how you meet recognized standards such as the Academy of Medical Educators (AoME) professional standards (AoME 2014).
	Within a clinical role: Consult colleagues, or refer patient to colleagues, as this is in the patient's best interests	As a community pediatrician you see a complex case and refer onto specialist Autism Spectrum Disorder services.
	Provide effective treatments based on the best available evidence	Example of prescribing off licence. The example of a 25-year-old patient demanding Melatonin for insomnia. The British National Formulary indicates only licenced for adults 55 years and over.
	Avoid providing medical care to yourself or anyone with whom you have a close personal relationship	Saying no to a close colleague who asked you to prescribe Diazepam for them
1.3 Record your work clearly, accurately and legibly	Make records at the same time as the events you are recording or as soon as possible after	At out-patients the clinic case notes are not available and the online system was down. You wrote notes on a loose piece of paper and have lost them and you couldn't remember the treatment plan.

Source: Adapted from GMC (2020).

Table 6.2 Domain 2: Safety and quality.

Attributes	Examples of principles and values	Examples of content
2.1 Contribute to and comply with systems to protect patients	Take part in systems of quality assurance and quality improvement Reviewing patient feedback Report suspected adverse drug reactions	Undertake a quality improvement project with your team to improve monitoring of blood sugar levels. Using patient feedback to then improve written information regarding side-effects of medication. Implement a process in your department to identify and report any suspected side-effects and audit the impact.
2.2 Respond to risks to safety	Report risks in the health care environment to your employing or contracting bodies Ask for advice when you have concerns that a colleague is not fit to practice Offer help in emergencies in clinical settings	A serious adverse event occurred due to lack of agreed procedures in the department. A colleague that you believe is drinking alcohol on duty denies this when you approach him. Escalated for advice to clinical director and your defense body. As a trainee in medicine you offered to cover ITU shifts.
2.3 Risks posed by your health	Be immunized against common serious communicable diseases where vaccines are available	Be the first to offer to have the COVID vaccine and make it known to all colleagues and patients.

Source: Adapted from GMC (2020).

Table 6.3 Domain 3: Communication, partnership and teamwork.

Attributes	Examples of principles and values	Examples of content
3.1 Communicate effectively	Must listen to patients, take account of their views, and respond honestly to their questions	Providing support for the parents of a 10-year-old patient with cystic fibrosis.
3.2 Work collaboratively with colleagues	Must treat colleagues fairly and with respect	Describing how you attempted to resolve issues between colleagues in an MDT.
	Must be aware of how your behavior may influence others within and outside the team	Reflecting on feedback from an Advanced Nurse Practitioner stating that you are a good role model for the entire clinical team.
3.3 Teaching, training supporting and assessing	Must make sure that all staff you manage have appropriate supervision	Checking the competency level of a trainee by direct observation of their clinical skills.
	Be willing to take on a mentoring role for more junior doctors and other health care professionals	Volunteering to take on a mentoring role for a newly appointed consultant colleague.
3.4 Continuity and coordination of care	When you delegate the care of a patient to others, must ensure the person is competent	Delegating medicine reviews to a community pharmacist–observing the pharmacist directly to assure yourself they were competent.
3.5 Establish and maintain partnerships with patients	Treat patients with respect whatever their life choices and beliefs	Reflecting on a patient with severe asthma and diabetes refusing to have the COVID vaccine.

Source: Adapted from GMC (2020).

Table 6.4 Domain 4: Maintaining trust.

Attributes	Examples of principles and values	Examples of content
4.1 Show respect for patients	Be open and honest with patients if thing go wrong	Apologizing to a patient whose cancer screening was delayed due to a form going missing.
4.2 Treat patients and colleagues fairly and without discrimination	Should challenge a colleague treating another colleague with discrimination	After witnessing bullying you escalate this unprofessional behavior to your line manager.
	Have adequate indemnity cover so that a patient will not be disadvantaged if they claim about your clinical care	Due to lack of clarity about what was covered by NHS indemnity in your NHS role you take out extended cover with a private provider.
4.3 Act with honesty and integrity	Co-operate with formal inquiries and complaints	Being asked to provide a detailed explanation of a claim of inadequate assessment of a patient in the Emergency Department.
	Honest and trustworthy when writing reports– make sure that any documents you sign are not misleading	Undertaking an audit of all Personal Income Payment (PIP) forms for a 12-month period to check accuracy.

Source: Adapted from GMC (2020).

Examples of Reflective Entries

This next section provides a series of examples of reflective entries. There are many formats and toolkits available to use. Some formats work better for some individual doctors, and in other scenarios there is an expectation to follow a prescribed model. A useful resource is the joint Academy of Medical Royal Colleges (AoMRC) and the Conference of Postgraduate Deans (COPMeD) reflective practice toolkit (Academy of Medical Royal Colleges and the Conference of Postgraduate Deans 2018). We have used a simple format of the event, reflection, action taken and outcome where appropriate (Tables 6.5–6.29).

Table 6.5 Consultant and clinical director, internal medicine.

Event

I had been working as a Consultant in acute medicine for five years and due to retirements I became the most "senior" in the department. I was asked to take on the role of interim Clinical Director. I went to fortnightly CD briefings from the Medical Director and other executives.

Reflection

I fairly soon began to think that I was out of my depth. I understood my own department well but soon realized that I knew very little about leadership, budgeting, business case writing and the politics outside of the hospital. I spoke to my unit MD and she advised I go on the leadership program in my region for newly appointed Clinical Directors. This made things worse and I began to get increasingly anxious in meetings. I realized that I needed to allow myself time to get to know the wider trust and learn new skills, but my performance in meetings that I chaired was getting worse. I felt I needed to be more aware of when I start to feel stressed. When stressed I am aware that I can move to a binary decision-making which reduces my performance.

Action

A colleague mentioned a one-day training course with the aim of enhancing personal resilience. This was delivered by a private company organized by our local postgraduate department. I was quite skeptical but thought I would give it a try. The focus of this training was on practical things to improve emotional awareness. I attended the EI training as I wanted to explore these tactics and others in more detail. I found the Box Breathing a particularly useful way for me to almost instantly relax and reduce my pulse rate.

Outcome

I now take more time to prepare for management meetings and when I feel that I am getting stressed I leave the meeting for 5–10 minutes and do box breathing exercises. If I am in a meeting where I cannot easily leave (e.g. if I am chairing), I will do Jacobson type muscle tensing and relaxing in my seat.

I find that the fact I know that these simple techniques are there for me and are effective also helps me to remain calm. I have encouraged all my direct reports and others to explore mindfulness-type exercises and learning.

Links to GMC Domains

Domain 1: Knowledge, Skills and Performance – competent in all aspects of your work including management

Domain 3: Communication, Partnership and Teamwork – be aware of how your behavior may influence others within and outside the team

Potential supporting documents that might be included:

• Training session program with stated learning objectives.
• Anonymized copies of mail/correspondence to direct reports.

Table 6.6 General practitioner out of hours.

Event

I saw an 18-month-old child on a home visit out of hours. The child presented with abdominal pain and diarrhea. I was put under a lot of pressure from the father, who appeared under the influence of alcohol, to admit the patient. Although the child didn't need admission, reluctantly I agreed. The patient was admitted to hospital unnecessarily and despite this, the aggressive father was still not placated.

Reflection

I felt the situation was beyond my control and possibly not dealt with effectively. I thought that I needed to examine my techniques in dealing with a verbally aggressive relative.

Action

The out-of-hours provider was running a half-day session on "aggression in the consultation and how to deal with it," so I attended. This was very valuable and in a way cathartic in that I was able to listen to others and their experiences. The main thing I gained was a sense of not being alone in having this type of experience.

In the workshop sessions my admission of the child was seen as a good option as it put myself and the child in a position of safety. I did however pick up that the way in which I initially dealt with the father probably reflected his anger back on him and possibly inflamed the situation. The father had met me at the door and said "my son needs to be in hospital and you need to admit him" I replied with something like "give me a chance to see him first" which probably set the tone. I learned that being seen to accept the relative's concern may have diffused the situation and that using body language to "tone down" the aggression is important. In the situation I had responded to the aggression with aggression. I will try to use these techniques in future and will record them as they arise.

Links to GMC Domains

Domain 1: Knowledge, Skills and Performance – competent in all aspects of your work.

Domain 2: Safety and Quality – take prompt action if you think patient safety may be seriously compromised.

Potential supporting documents that might be included:

• Learning objectives/agenda for the workshop.
• Any feedback from the workshop.

Table 6.7 Specialty doctor in anesthetics.

Event

I run a tertiary pain clinic along with a clinical psychologist. I had seen a male patient on numerous occasions over a couple of years. He had a number of remedial operations for a prolapsed disc. I was aware the patient had become increasingly dissatisfied with his care and treatment. At the next out-patients (via VC) I decided to advice Pregabalin for neuropathic pain and informed the patient about the side-effects and target symptoms.

Table 6.7 (Continued)

At the next clinic the patient was very angry as there had been no response and the patient accused me of stating that the response would be 100%. As the conversation went on the patient disclosed that he had recorded the last consultation and therefore had proof that I had promised a 100% response rate.
Reflection
I was initially angry with the patient. I was quite shocked that he had recorded my consultation. I got advice from my defense union and the BMA. I was shocked to hear that in law the patient's consultation is treated as the patient's personal information and they can do whatever they wish with it. I reflected on this and realized that the patient's behavior was borne out of frustration that no treatments had ever worked.
Action
I now routinely tell patients at the beginning of each session that I will write with a summary of the discussion. I send a letter summarizing details of the management plan. Patient feedback on these letters has been very positive and other colleagues across the hospital are now doing the same.
Links to GMC Domains
Domain 1: Knowledge, Skills and Performance – competent in all aspects of your work; applying knowledge and experience to practice.
Domain 3: Communication, Partnership and Teamwork – working in partnership with patients.
Potential supporting documents that might be included:
• Feedback from patients regarding the summary letters.
• Copy of anonymized summary letter.

Table 6.8 Things going really well – consultant in obstetrics.

Event
I was on Delivery Suite duty and had a phone call from one of the midwifes regarding a patient. I have worked with this midwife for years and consider her a skilled clinician and good decision-maker. The fetal heart rate had one spike and she was concerned as the mother was getting increasing anxious and hadn't started dilation. I decided to go and assess the mum and baby. Mum was 18, first baby with no partner or support. I scanned and kept an eye on fetal heart rate. I sat with mum with the midwife and we jointly discussed options. One option of course was a Cesarean section if the baby was in distress. The heart rate deteriorated immediately after that and 20 minutes later mum was in theater, with epidural, and I operated quickly but calmly, talking to mum as I went along.
All went well with no complications and the baby's Apgar score was maximum on delivery. Three hours later I did a quick ward round and mum thanked me for everything I had done.

(Continued)

Table 6.8 (Continued)

Reflection

I reflected later that this was a good outcome as a result of good teamwork and how lucky I am to have such good skilled colleagues. This reminded me of the importance of team working. When the focus is the patients, mum and baby, then we get good outcomes.

Action

I have made a conscious effort to offer a verbal thank you to any colleagues who are doing their job well. I follow this up with a personal e-mail. I recognize that we are all too often critical of each other and the system in which we work.

Links to GMC Domains

Domain 3: Communication, Partnership and Teamwork – work collaboratively with colleagues, respecting their skills and contributions.

Potential supporting documents that might be included:

• Example of anonymized thank you emails.

Table 6.9 A general practitioner in a training role.

Event

I have been a GP trainer for 10 years. I am recognized as an advanced trainer because of my experience and skills. I have an ST3 trainee on placement now. From day one he had been argumentative with all staff including myself. He would not follow advice or direction. I took the usual steps to help him improve his performance and confidence, including 30-minute consultations, 50% under direct supervision, videoed consultations and case-based discussions.

I completed the educational supervisor's report six weeks ago with the trainee face-to-face. He got extremely angry and stormed out the room, and has written a series of e-mails to the local deanery office complaining about me personally and claiming the practice should be shut down.

Reflection

This was the most challenging trainee I have ever tried to help. My initial reflections were that he had either mental health issues in his personal life and/or it may have been that he couldn't cope with the huge diversity of problems you see as a GP. I then got feedback from the deanery office that the trainee had been arrested for dealing in illegal drugs and was under investigation by the GMC.

I was initially surprised to hear this news. I wasn't sure from the limited feedback I had whether that meant he was using drugs himself. If so, I had missed that and so had all colleagues in the practice. Had we been blinded by his arrogant and aggressive demeanor?

Action

As a group of four GP trainers we have agreed that one of us will act as purely mentor/pastoral support for any trainees on placement with us. This is in addition to the normal support we would offer. Our hope is that this additional level might encourage trainees to disclose any issues that could be affecting their performance.

Table 6.9 (Continued)

Links to GMC Domains

Domain 1: Knowledge, Skills and Performance – must be competent in all aspects of your work, including...teaching.

Domain 3: Communication, Partnership and Teamwork – honest and objective when assessing the performance of colleagues.

Potential supporting documents that might be included:

• Anonymized extract from the educational supervisor's report.

• Anonymized extracts from e-mail from the trainee.

Table 6.10 Consultant obstetrician – feedback from a lecture.

Event

I do a regular lecture on prenatal eclampsia to medical students from the local medical school as a part of their obstetrics and gynecology rotation. This was normally a one-hour lecture. I had used the same slides for a number of years and I usually reviewed them a few days before in case our local protocol has been revised, but it is essentially the same lecture that I have given for a few years and the feedback has generally been ok. Because of COVID the face-to-face lecture was changed to a webinar.

On the day, I couldn't work the slide show and the internet kept cutting off and when it came back the slides had disappeared and I took ages to find them and share with the online audience. I found myself getting flustered and annoyed. I muted my mike and phoned the medical school administrator but her phone went to answerphone. I keep going despite all the glitches. The feedback from the students was so poor that the administrator rang me the next day to tell me.

Reflections

I reflected on her comments and rang her back to say that it was my own fault as I hadn't prepared or rehearsed the system and asked if someone could give me some technical training.

Action

I shared my experience with colleagues at the end of one of our weekly MDTs and a few said they were in the same boat. A month later the local Postgraduate office set up a two-hour session, and there were about 40 different professionals there. I learnt that delivering a webinar required different skills and more interaction than a face-to-face lecture. We got advice on how to structure a webinar, such as sending out the slides beforehand and using Q and A sessions in the middle.

Outcome

Feedback from the next cohort was a lot better and I now enjoy using the technology to try and engage the students in their own learning, and I am less stressed.

Links to GMC Domains

Domain 1: Knowledge, Skills and Performance – competent in all aspects of your work including...teaching.

Domain 3: Communication, Partnership and Teamwork – be prepared to contribute to teaching and training doctors and students.

Potential supporting documents that might be included:

• Copy of initial feedback from the students.

• Copy of the training session agenda–including learning objectives and any assessment.

• Copy of further feedback from students.

Table 6.11 General practitioner – asthma management plan.

Event

One of my colleagues referred a patient I normally review to the local asthma clinic. The letter from the consultant in respiratory medicine was critical of the care being provided to the patient, suggesting that the care plan was inadequate with the patient only prescribed one inhaler.

I reviewed this patient's case notes and was relieved to see that I had prescribed three inhalers, but that he had only obtained the Ventolin and not the other two. I called the patient on the telephone to review. The patient said that he only liked taking the Ventolin as the other two inhalers made him feel sick and he felt they didn't work.

Reflection

I realized that although I had discussed a personalized management plan for the asthma, I hadn't really explored the patient's view of his inhalers. It was also clearer that the patient didn't understand the importance of the escalation plan if he had an attack.

I realized that I needed to be more systematic in my approach to asthma plans and not to assume anything.

Action

I brought up this case at one of our practice meetings. We agreed that we needed to use the skills of a community pharmacist that we could access from the local GP cluster. This would enable us to have more monitoring over asthma plans and the starting point would be an audit. We also agreed to devise a patient pathway so that we would be more consistent in our use of the practice asthma nurse more often.

Links to GMC Domains

Domain 1: Knowledge, Skills and Performance – be competent in all aspects of your work/keep professional knowledge and skills up to date.

Domain 2: Safety and Quality – take part in regular review and audits of your work.

Domain 3: Communication, Partnership and Teamwork – must listen to patients, take account of their views.

Potential supporting documents that might be included:

• Anonymized letter from the respiratory consultant.
• Summary of more recent audit cycle.

Table 6.12 A thank you – associate specialist in adult psychiatry.

Event

I assessed a new patient, a 20-year-old single man. He presented with a 3-month history of auditory hallucinations that were becoming increasing distressing for him. The patient was calm but worried about these experiences.

He didn't meet ICD-10 criteria for schizophrenia but it was clear in my view that he was developing a psychotic illness.

Table 6.12 (Continued)

I explained to the patient that I thought he had early signs of a psychotic illness. He became very tearful at this point. I explained how common these experiences are. He eventually asked if I was going to lock him up in the local mental hospital. This was clearly a major concern for him. I reassured him that most patients with these experiences respond well to treatment and do not need to go into hospital at all. I prescribed olanzapine at night and planned to review him in three weeks. When next seen he was a lot better. On leaving he handed me an envelope with a thank-you letter in it. In this he thanked me for being understanding, calm and reassuring. His biggest worry was being locked up forever in a hospital.

Reflection

This patient's feedback reminded me of the need to treat and manage every patient as an individual. I reflected that there were no easy-read information sheets for patients with first episode psychosis, and that if I looked on the internet there was so much misinformation if you didn't know where to look.

Action

I drafted a leaflet and asked this patient to sense-check it. This is now given out to all patients, but also forms the basis of the verbal advice offered.

Links to GMC Domains

Domain 1: Knowledge, Skills and Performance.

Domain 2: Safety and Quality.

Domain 3: Communication, Partnership and Teamwork – listen to patients, take account of their views.

Potential supporting documents that might be included:

• Copy of thank-you letter.
• Copy of patient information leaflet.

Table 6.13 Issue with authorship of a study – consultant cardiologist.

Event

I was Principle Investigator for a study exploring the outcomes from different approaches to stents. There is a team of four of us as researchers. We got funding from a national charity and all four were named as authors. We have a busy research unit in the department. We had an editorial meeting four months ago, which I chaired, and a colleague who is a Reader in Medicine turned up as if he was a co-author and had been involved. He does work in the lab but was not directly involved in this study. The meeting was very awkward and I closed it early and asked to speak with this colleague.

I got HR and legal advice and checked national guidance. I met with my colleague with HR present and checked his expectations. He stated that he wanted to be named on the study. He didn't give any real reason apart from saying he works in the lab. I spoke with the Department Head who just said in a very offhand way to just agree with him as he can be very awkward and best to keep him on side.

(Continued)

Table 6.13 (Continued)

Reflection

I reflected on the position I was in. This colleague had not been involved in any aspect of the work and so I could not in all consciousness agree to name him. I knew this would displease my Head of Department but I felt I had to do the right thing.

Action

I mailed my colleague copying in HR and the Head of Department stating that he would not be named as author as he had not been involved in any aspect of the study, and to do so would be in breach of guidelines. I drafted a protocol and presented it at a departmental meeting. This described the rules of authorship and a simple form to be completed at the beginning of any study naming the authors involved and what each role would be in the study.

Links to GMC Domains

Domain 1: Knowledge, Skills and Performance – competent in all aspects of your work including...research.

Domain 4: Maintaining trust – act with honesty and integrity when designing, organizing or carrying out research, and follow national research governance guidelines.

Potential supporting documents that might be included:

- Copy of protocol.
- Minutes of departmental meeting.
- Copy of anonymized mail to colleague.

Table 6.14 General practitioner – missed diagnosis.

Event

I saw a 45-year-old woman with a long history of tension headache. She presented to surgery three times over a three-week period with the same symptoms. I saw her for the previous attendances and her presentation I thought was the same as before. She was a vague historian and inconsistent in her description of her symptoms.

I ordered routine bloods, not expecting any different findings. The ESR was 120 mm/h. I arranged to see the patient urgently that afternoon. She had loss of temporal pulse but no obvious thickening of the artery.

Refection

I realized I had missed Giant cell arteritis. I shared this with the patient and apologized that I had not picked it up on earlier. I initiated treatment and explained risks of blindness. The patient appeared reassured.

I realized that I had not explored a wide enough differential and because of the patient's history of tension and non-specific headaches, I assumed that was the case. I didn't explore the symptoms and wasn't proactive enough in ordering blood tests.

Table 6.14 (Continued)

Action

I personally undertook an audit of those patients currently diagnosed with
headache of any cause. I revisited the local protocol from the neurology
department on assessment and management of headache. I presented the
results at a local training session with colleagues. I then developed a simple
algorithm to ensure that as a practice it is less likely that we miss potentially
serious causes of headache.

Links to GMC Domains

Domain 1: Knowledge, Skills and Performance – must be familiar with guidelines
and developments that affect your work.

Domain 2: Safety and Quality – taking part in audit.

Domain 4: Maintaining trust – honest and open with patients when things go
wrong.

Potential supporting documents that might be included:

• Summary of audit findings.
• Copy of headache algorithm.

Table 6.15 ST6 doctor in training in medicine.

Event

I was on call in the Medical Assessment Unit and also covering the ED for any
emergencies. I reviewed a 30-year-old fit man c/o breathlessness, no wheeze,
tired and drained otherwise, nothing else. On physical examination the only
finding of note was creps lower right side. Temperature was 37.8, pulse 85,
breaths 16 per min.

I ordered a chest X-ray, FBC and U and Es. I wasn't expecting much to come
back as abnormal. Then there was an arrest in the ED, which took two hours.
Unfortunately, the patient passed away and I had to speak to the woman's
husband. After that I needed a break and stopped for a quick coffee for
15 minutes. When I arrived back on the Medical Assessment Unit the nurse in
charge asked me to see the 30-year man again. He looked ill, temp was 38.8,
pulse 115, BR 24. Immediately I thought of sepsis secondary to chest infection.
I started IV antibiotics and followed the MAU protocol. Four hours later the
patient was improving and he stabilized.

Reflection.

At the end of my shift I sat with another trainee I know well. I shared with her
that I thought I should have considered sepsis earlier and this patient was a
near-miss. I decided that I must have a high index of suspicion even in patients
like this who are in the low-risk group, young, fit and healthy.

Action

The first thing I did was to present this case at the department MDT a few weeks
later. I wanted to share my experience and to highlight the need to constantly
consider sepsis as a diagnosis. I then undertook an audit of the last 12 months
of admissions with a diagnosis of sepsis and reviewed all the case notes. This
helped me to revise our MAU protocol.

(Continued)

Table 6.15 (Continued)

Links to GMC Domains

Domain 1: Knowledge, Skills and Performance – must be familiar with guidelines and developments that affect your work.

Domain 2: Safety and Quality – taking part in audit.

Domain 4: Maintaining trust – honest and open with patients when things go wrong.

Potential supporting documents that might be included:
- Summary of audit findings.
- Copy of revised protocol.

Table 6.16 ST5 in geriatric medicine–confusing DNACPRs.

Event

I had just started working on a 20-bedded female ward for elderly care. Most patients had various levels of dementia and were very frail. I decided to review all the case notes and a part of that was cross-checking DNACPR paperwork. I noticed there were two patients with the same forename and family name and born in the same year. I paid particular attention to these case notes as I had in the last year been given the wrong case notes for a patient attending clinic and only realized 10 minutes into the consultation.

I noticed there were 4 separate and different DNACPR forms in each set of notes and I was confused as to which was whose. I checked with the senior nurse on with me that day and we both looked at the directions. He cross-checked with a summary sheet on the ward office but we were still confused.

Reflection

I need to check and recheck patient ID as a routine. On this occasion we had spotted the mix-up but this was a near miss waiting to happen.

Action

With the two patients in question the consultant and myself reviewed the decision with each patient and their families and the documentation was clear. I also audited all elderly wards with two colleagues across the trust – a total of 10 wards. We found two cases of incomplete paperwork that may have led to confusion in the event of an arrest. This led us to revise the review process in line with national guidance.

Links to GMC Domains

Domain 1: Knowledge, Skills and Performance – must be familiar with guidelines and developments that affect your work.

Domain 2: Safety and Quality – taking part in audit.

Potential supporting documents that might be included:
- Summary of audit findings.
- Copy of revised process for checking DNACPR decisions.

Table 6.17 General practitioner – a compliment.

Event

I had been involved in the initial diagnosis of 10-year-old boy with bone cancer. He then went into the oncology service but I kept oversight through letters from the oncology and surgery teams looking after him. I rang the family every month or so just to check on how things were and to offer any help they needed. The Macmillan nurse was the key worker and I really didn't have an active role in the boy's treatment.

The nurse rang me about six months ago to inform me that a recent scan had showed multiple secondaries in both lungs and the prognosis was poor. The parents had been informed and they had told their son. I rang the parents that evening at the end of surgery to say I had heard the news. The mother was crying and upset. I spoke to her for about 10 minutes and she calmed down.

The boy unfortunately passed away four weeks after that at home. One of my colleagues did the death certificate. A month after that I received a thank-you card from the parents. In it they thanked me for my support and they said that they knew if their son needed me that I was there for them and just knowing that was a huge comfort to them.

Reflection

This reminded me of the importance of that human interaction and making patients and relatives aware that you care, and are available but without intruding too much. It reminded me of one of the main reasons I went into medicine and into General Practice in particular.

Action

At our Balint group I reflected on this family and the team echoed my own thoughts. We agreed that we should make it part of day-to-day practice to identify patients and relatives that we don't clinically need to see because of receiving specialist services elsewhere in the system, to remind them that we are there for them if needed. I also undertook a review of caseloads and devised a system of flagging patients under care of cancer services in the first instance.

Links to GMC Domains

Domain 3: Communication, partnership and teamwork – work collaboratively with colleagues, respecting their skills and contributions/be readily accessible to patients.

Potential supporting documents that might be included:

- Copy of the thank-you card.
- Copy of review of case notes.
- Copy of revised protocol for ringing patients/relatives.

Table 6.18 General practice trainee – a missed fracture.

Event

I had only been working in the Emergency Department for two weeks but had done acute medicine for six months on my rotation and felt fairly confident. I was at the end of a very busy night shift. We had had a major RTC and two arrests. My last patient was a 24-year-old male cyclist who had fallen off his bicycle about 36 hours previously. On examination he had tenderness on the dorsum of his left hand but no significant swelling. He had full movement and no evidence of neurological damage. I ordered an X-ray. Within 20 minutes the pictures were available. I couldn't see anything obvious and decided to let the patient go home and advised paracetamol for analgesia. As I was fairly sure he didn't have a fracture, I didn't organize for him to return to the fracture clinic.

My next shift was two days later. The consultant on with me asked to have a chat. She explained I had missed a fracture of the scaphoid but that the formal radiology report picked it up and the patient had been seen in clinic and a cast put on.

Reflection

This was a reminder to me that I must follow guidelines in the department so that any queried fracture must be referred to the next day's fracture clinic and if in any doubt to put a back slab on. I also reflected that I was working outside of my competency level as I was inexperienced in spotting possible fractures such as the scaphoid.

Action

During the rest of my time in the ED I sought out experienced clinicians skilled in reporting X-rays and got them to test and retest my skills. I undertook a wide range of WPBAs and as a result felt more confident in reporting images in general.

Links to GMC Domains

Domain 1: Knowledge, Skills and Performance – recognize and work within the limits of your competence.

Potential supporting documents that might be included:

• Copies of WPBAs with feedback from various supervisors.

Table 6.19 Specialty doctor in general medicine.

Event

I was doing a busy general medical clinic. There was a wide range of conditions, but there were a lot of lower GI patients. I saw a 45-year-old male patient with a diagnosis of ulcerative colitis. This was the third time I had seen this patient in the last four months. This appointment had been expedited at the request of the GP who was concerned about the patient's weight loss.

The patient complained of recurrent cramps with no blood loss with weight loss of about a stone in that last three months, but I couldn't see his weight recorded in the notes for his last four appointments. The patient talked about being under stress due to being suspended from his job. I assumed this stress had exacerbated his ulcerative colitis and I advised him to increase the dose of his usual treatment.

Table 6.19 (Continued)

I asked the F2 to do a physical examination and order bloods. The screen came back with anemia, a picture of GI bleeding and a raised ESR. A scan confirmed the diagnosis of stage 3 cancer in the transverse colon.
Reflection
I had missed a cancer diagnosis. If I had taken the history of weight loss more seriously I may have been more proactive. I put his symptoms down to the ulcerative colitis. The lesson for me was to be more proactive and not make assumptions. I thought as well that I should not let previous diagnoses color what might be a new presentation. The missed weight recordings was another factor.
Action
The first thing I needed to do was to meet the patient and apologize. I was very nervous about this but the patient was so reassuring and thanked me for "putting up" with him at clinic. I also triggered a meeting with senior admin of the OPD to look at how we record measurements that don't go through our online system, such as temperature and weight. We devised a simple checklist that was stapled to the front of all clinical notes. I undertook a quick review of the clinical profile of the clinics and we decided to establish a specialist lower GI clinic and to run those with our surgical and endoscopy colleagues.
Links to GMC Domains
Domain 2: Safety and Quality – taking part in regular reviews and audits of your work.
Domain 4: Maintaining trust – open and honest with patients if things go wrong...and offer an apology.
Potential supporting documents that might be included:
• Copy of physical health measurement checklist.
• Copy of review of case mix in the generic clinic.

Table 6.20 Consultant in general pediatrics – timing of ward rounds.

Event
My timings of my ward rounds were not set in stone. They happened at different times across the week due to pressure on me to attend at the assessment unit where the trainees are less experienced and constantly calling me on the phone for advice or requesting consultant presence to further assess patients. This system of flexible timing I felt worked well.
We then had a not-unexpected death on the ward– a female patient aged 14 with quite complex cystic fibrosis and cardiac anomaly. I spoke to the parents after the child passed and they were distressed, but thanked me and all the staff for caring for their daughter. About threeweeks after that the unit received a letter of complaint from the family basically saying that a major issue for them was lack of access to me, as the ward rounds were held at various random times.

(Continued)

Table 6.20 (Continued)

Reflection

I reflected on their comments and spoke with the two ward managers and other
staff. They all fed back that it was frustrating for them and no doubt for
families as there was no scheduled time in the week when parents could speak
to me. The nurses in particular had been fielding demands from parents to
speak to me. They would often make excuses for me saying that I was very
busy elsewhere in the hospital. I realized this was inappropriate and I had to
take action myself.

Action

I discussed a new consultant rota with colleagues. The issue was to provide cover
for the assessment unit. We redeployed an advanced nurse practitioner from
the ward to cover the assessment unit. I now have my ward rounds at fixed
times in the week, and devised an information leaflet giving times that families
could meet with me.

Links to GMC Domains

Domain 3: Communication, Partnership and Teamwork – be considerate to those
close to the patient and be sensitive and responsive in giving them information
and support.

Domain 4: Maintaining trust – be open and honest with patients if things go
wrong, put matters right.

Potential supporting documents that might be included:
• Letter of complaint.
• Copy of new consultant rota.
• Copy of relatives' information leaflet.

Table 6.21 Doctor in training in surgery – a gift.

Event

I clerked a 67-year-old man when I was on take. He had a confirmed diagnosis of
bowel cancer. I spent some time with his wife and son, both of whom were
very worried. I assisted in theater where unfortunately the patient arrested and
after two days in ITU he died.

About a month after this death I received a letter from the family with a cheque
for £500. The note from the patient's wife thanked me for all I had done for
her husband, and that he had wanted me to have something.

Reflection

My initial reaction was of shock and surprise. I thought that I was just doing my
job but was pleased at a personal level. To be honest I started to think what I
might spend the money on. Then I remembered there was Trust guidance on
gifts and I checked it on the internet.

Action

I send the cheque back to the family thanking them. I suggested that they could
donate the money to Cancer UK or a similar charity.

Links to GMC Domains

Domain 4: Maintaining trust – Honesty in financial dealings.

Potential supporting documents that might be included:
• Copy of thank-you letter.
• Copy of your reply and evidence of transfer of the money.

Table 6.22 Consultant dermatologist – medical education qualification.

Event

I was asked to take on a lead role for revising the teaching approach for years 4
and 5 in my local medical school. I had worked as an Honorary Senior Lecturer
for a number of years, delivering teaching in medicine and dermatology in
particular.

Reflection

I recognized that although I had a lot of experience in learning and teaching, my
theoretical basis wasn't as strong as it could be, and this new role required a
high level of understanding and educational pedagogy.

Action

I am studying a Master's in Medical Education from my local University and am
currently undertaking the research element exploring CPD models of
leadership with consultants in a nearby Trust. Through working to diploma
level in formal studying pushed me to a higher level of understanding of
educational theory (and theory into practice), particularly assessment which is
key to my day job. In addition, I have focused on CPD models and the lack of
CPD for formal medical leaders.

Outcome

I have embedded my learning into day-to-day practice and have moved from
lectures as knowledge transfer processes to small group work and workshops
with very specific learning objectives. I have also migrated this learning into
so-called non-learning environments. For example, I now am very clear that
with any new initiative the scoping has to start with: "what are the outcomes
we wish to see?" This I feel has enabled me to become more efficient in
managing the team.

Recognizing that my day-to-day practice has changed, I have encouraged all
senior staff that I line-manage to consider a similar qualification at an early
stage in their career.

Links to GMC Domains

Domain 1: Knowledge, Skills and Performance – competent in all aspects of your
work including...teaching.

Domain 3: Communication, partnership and teamwork – be prepared to
contribute to teaching and training doctors and students.

Potential supporting documents that might be included:

- Academic transcript.
- Qualification certificates.
- If dissertation element–include Research protocol.
- Feedback from students.

Table 6.23 Consultant in adult psychiatry – complaint from patient.

Event

I assessed a patient as a second opinion. The patient was subject to criminal court proceedings and social services were involved. I interviewed the patient twice and reviewed all past case notes. The patient was insisting that his diagnosis was Bipolar Affective Disorder and that he wanted medication for that. On review he had been diagnosed with a Personality Disorder 15 years beforehand, and although bipolar was considered, it was stated clearly by four different consultants and a clinical psychologist who saw him at the time that there was no evidence to support a diagnosis of bipolar.

I shared my opinion with the patient that his diagnosis was a personality disorder and there was no evidence of bipolar. He instantly became very angry and verbally abusive. He repeatedly shouted that he had bipolar and wanted medication. The patient eventually stormed out of the room. A week later I received a letter of complaint accusing me of being abusive and unprofessional.

Reflection

I reflected on my approach to this patient. I did wonder whether I had been too abrupt when I shared my opinion in regard to his diagnosis. He clearly had the firm belief that he had a bipolar disorder and this is what he expected and wanted to be told. In the context of a busy clinic, perhaps I hadn't taken his firm expectations into account.

Action

After reflecting on this, my medical secretary now sends out an opt-in letter for all patients. I have added a simple paper-based questionnaire asking the patient their expectations of attending the clinic. There are just six questions. Patients are asked to bring it with them when they first attend. If they don't they are asked to fill it out by reception staff as they arrive at the unit before being seen. This is then used as a starting point to explore their hopes and expectations.

Links to GMC Domains

Domain 1: Knowledge, Skills and Performance – competent in all aspects of your work.

Domain 3: Communication, partnership and teamwork – listen to patients, take account of their views.

Potential supporting documents that might be included:

• Anonymized copy of complaint letter.
• Anonymized copy of evidence of discussion of expectations from patients.
• Feedback from patients on their view of the usefulness of the questionnaire.

Table 6.24 General practitioner – complaint from relatives.

Event

I had seen a male patient on and off for over 15 years. He was now in his 60s and had suffered with lower back pain for years. He had had a number of operations and remedial surgery, but continued to have lower pain across L2/3.

I had referred him to the practice physiotherapist and also to a private osteopath. The local MSK service were still seeing him, but it was clear to me that there was no surgical or other intervention that was likely to help.

I reviewed him regularly over two to three months, mainly to try and rationalize his polypharmacy. He had been on increasing doses of Diazepam and he had disclosed to me that on occasions he was buying some top-up on the street. I spent some time with him and we agreed a withdrawal program over a number of months, reducing the dose very slowly.

The practice received a letter of complaint from his wife about a month after starting the withdrawal. The patient had actually only reduced the dose by 1 mg, so shouldn't be experiencing any withdrawal effects yet. His wife accused me of insisting that he stopped the Diazepam and that he was getting "worse by the hour."

I saw the patient with his wife the week I got the letter. After a lengthy session it transpired that the patient had been buying up to 50 mg of Diazepam on a daily basis and using this with the prescribed 20 mg daily. His usual supply of street drug had disappeared and he was in withdrawal.

Reflection

When I reflected it was clear that I hadn't explored his street drug usage in enough detail. Also I hadn't involved his wife in the decision at any point. I know the family well and it would have been easy to invite her in to explain the situation. If I had done that, she would have been able to encourage the patient to disclose the true extent of street usage.

Action

There were a number of lessons for me with this patient. The first was that we devised a simple protocol to ensure that any patient on any withdrawal program is asked if we can speak to family members before finalizing the plan. Another was that I needed to refresh and update my knowledge about street/illegal drugs. I contacted the local community drugs team and arranged to sit in with some of their clinics on a Thursday afternoon over four weeks.

Links to GMC Domains

Domain 1: Knowledge, Skills and Performance – competent in all aspects of your work.

Domain 3: Communication, partnership and teamwork – listen to patients, take account of their views.

Potential supporting documents that might be included:

• Copy of new protocol.
• Reflections on new knowledge from attending the local drugs team.

Table 6.25 Consultant histopathologist/sub-dean.

Event

Over the last six months there have been a number of trainees coming to me asking about training in quality improvement (QI), as some of Trusts in the region had implemented a number of QI projects and they wanted trainees with QI experience to sit on various steering groups. This was really good management and leadership experience for the trainees to get. I recognized that we needed to provide all trainees with learning opportunities to enhance their quality improvement skills to ensure safer and improved services for patients. I set up a new role of Associate Dean (AD) for QI skills training for all trainees and appointed a highly qualified individual to this part-time role.

Reflection

Through the supervision of the AD it became clear that barriers existed within the NHS to quality improvement, and one of these is that some consultants and GPs do not recognize the need and hence are not appropriate role models for trainees.

Action

We have started a series of roadshows across the patch to target trainers regarding the importance of QI skills training. In addition, we have brokered a QI strategy across all the Trusts in the region. These initiatives will enable trainees to gain access to high quality training in improvement science mapped to the Generic Professional Capabilities.

Links to GMC Domains

Domain 1: Knowledge, Skills and Performance – competent in all aspects of your work, including management/teaching.

Domain 3: Communication, partnership and teamwork – contribute to teaching and training doctors and students.

Potential supporting documents that might be included:

- AD job description.
- Anonymized feedback from QI roadshow attendees.

Table 6.26 Associate Medical Director – escalation of concerns.

Event

I had been Associate Medical Director for clinical governance in our Trust for four years. I was on part secondment from my previous role as unit medical director of one of the smaller hospitals. A political decision was made to merge us with a nearby trust. We had to go through the usual reorganization that happens in the NHS all the time. There were a number of formal meetings and effectively I had to put the case forward that I should be slotted into the new organization in my current role. The process included consultation meetings with the new CEO of the new Trust. The outcome was I was slotted into my substantive role as unit medical director and I had to give up the clinical governance role.

The new CEO and her senior team clearly had very negative views of our previous processes. A new director of clinical governance was appointed and all of the systems I had established were disbanded with no obvious replacements. I felt there were significant patient safety issues as a result. I asked to meet with the new director but was told that was not needed. The audit team I had developed was disbanded, and the Significant Event Assessment unit was to be reorganized.

Table 6.26 (Continued)

Reflection

This was a difficult position in many ways. I was disappointed that I was not offered the clinical governance role in the new organization, but the fact that there were no basic processes live was of concern. I had attempted to flag my concerns, but I was repeatedly told that it wasn't my role.

Action

I took advice from colleagues, the BMA, my defense union and the local GMC liaison officer. As a few weeks went by I felt I had no choice but to formally write to the chair of the Trust and copy in the GMC Director of Standards.

Links to GMC Domains

Domain 1: Knowledge, Skills and Performance – competent in all aspects of your work, including management.

Domain 2: Safety and quality – must take prompt action if you think patient safety is or may be seriously compromised.

Potential supporting documents that might be included:

• Copy of correspondence.

Table 6.27 Specialty doctor in Medicine – working incollaboration.

Event

Over the last 12 months I have noticed that there has been a series of patients attending clinic with multiple comorbidity with a common theme of a diagnosis of myalgia encephalomyelitis (ME). I have found it really difficult to tease apart symptoms of ME from other illnesses. The patients with ME seem very well informed and all were a member of an ME forum and/or some other support organization.

Reflection

I realized I really didn't have either the knowledge of recent studies into ME or clinical experience of comorbidities. I discussed this with my consultant and I started to explore if there were any services locally that I could use to update my understanding. I was told of a consultant physician in a nearby Trust who had a special interest in ME and had published widely in the subject.

Action

I made contact with the consultant and asked if I could attend and observe some of the ME clinics. This was a great experience and she was inspirational. I met the chairperson of the regional ME association support group and was invited along and got involved. Throughout this I started drafting a summary of everything I had learnt. This exercise enhanced my knowledge of the recent research. The consultant in ME suggested I publish this and I have submitted it to a journal.

This series of patients has taught me to reflect on my gaps and take steps to meet those needs.

Links to GMC Domains

Domain 1: Knowledge, Skills and Performance – competent in all aspects of your work.

Domain 3: Communication, partnership and teamwork – listen to patients, take account of their views.

Potential supporting documents that might be included:

• Copy of submitted manuscript.

Table 6.28 Surgeon – the care of chronic regional pain syndrome.

Event

Four months ago I received a very brief referral from a GP asking me to assess a 23-year-old man with chronic regional pain syndrome (CRPS) for amputation of his left leg. The GP stated that the case was complex and I was only being asked to check whether there were any contra-indications for surgery.

I assessed the patient in the presence of his parents who kept answering questions for the patient. Near the end of the consultation I asked the parents to leave the room for a few minutes so I could physically examine the patient. I had two nurse chaperones with me. The parents became defensive and then angry and initially refused to leave the room. Eventually they did. I found nothing in my physical examination that would increase risk of general anesthesia. I ordered some routine X-rays and bloods.

Reflections

I knew very little about CRPS. I was aware that occasionally amputation was a recognized intervention. I looked on the internet for any national guidance and saw that the RCP was the only college with a set of guidelines.

Action

I thought that I can't be the only one, and sent an e-mail to the consultant body in the Trust to see if anyone else was involved who had experience of CRPS. It transpired that a number of us had been asked to see the same male patient via various routes. It was also obvious from the e-mail conversations that nursing and physiotherapist colleagues had extensive experience. This triggered a professionals meeting so that we could coordinate any opinion/treatment. In this meeting it was agreed that we should develop a pathway for patients with CRPS across the Trust so that we could improve the service, avoid duplicated investigations, and have a more evidence-based service for patients.

Links to GMC Domains

Domain 1: Knowledge, Skills and Performance – competent in all aspects of your work.

Domain 3: Communication, partnership and teamwork – work collaboratively with colleagues, respecting their skills and contributions listen to patients, take account of their views.

Potential supporting documents that might be included:

- Copy of RCP guidance.
- Copy of e-mail conversations.
- Copy of new patient pathway.

Table 6.29 Consultant dermatologies – gender identity.

Event

I saw a patient at a routine dermatology clinic. The patient presented with severe psoriasis and was on hormones for gender reassignment. The patient appeared male, aged 24, sporting a full beard and was quite muscular. I asked the patient how he wanted to be addressed and he was unsure at the beginning but did say ..."I suppose I identify as female most of the time but it's 50/50." I advised the patient on treatment and wrote what I thought was a fairly standard letter back to the GP.

Four weeks later I had a letter back from the GP castigating me for referring to the patient as "he." I rang the GP that afternoon to check and it transpired that the GP had shown my letter to the patient who was extremely angry. I explained that it was an error but that the patient when I saw them was at best ambivalent about which pronoun they wanted used, but that of course it was my fault and I should have checked. I wrote to the patient explaining and offering an apology. I did not hear anything else.

Reflection

I now double-check with all patients what they prefer to be called and if any are unsure I say I just refer to the patient. In addition, I was aware that my knowledge and understanding of the care pathway for gender realignment was sketchy at best.

Action

I discussed this with my College mentor and after further refection I contacted the local Consultant Psychiatrist who leads on gender reassignment for the region. She was very helpful and when we met, she explained the latest care pathway and she shared all the protocols and guidance.

Links to GMC Domains

Domain 1: Knowledge, Skills and Performance – competent in all aspects of your work, be familiar with guidelines and developments that affect your work.

Domain 3: Communication, partnership and teamwork – listen to patients, take account of their views.

Domain 4: Maintaining trust – offer an apology.

Potential supporting documents that might be included:
• Copy of letter from GP.
• Copy of letter to the patient.

Chapter Summary

In this chapter we have provided details of the four domains in GMP, along with examples of principles and values with brief examples of possible content.

We have also provided a series of simple reflective narratives as examples as to how one might want to start to frame reflections, and the learning that was triggered by them.

References

Academy of Medical Educators (2014). Professional standards for medical, dental and veterinary educators (3rd edn). Layout 1. https://www.medicaleducators.org/Professional-Standards (accessed 16 May 2021).

Academy of Medical Royal Colleges and Conference of Postgraduate Medical Deans (2018). *Academy and COPMeD Reflective Practice Toolkit.* https://www.copmed.org.uk/images/docs/reflective_practice/Reflective_Practice_Toolkit.pdf (accessed 12 May 2021).

Chan, S.W., Tulloch, E., Cooper, E.S. et al. (2017). Montgomery and informed consent: where are we now? *British Medical Journal* **357**: j2224. https://doi.org/10.1136/bmj.j2224.

Dewey, J. (1938). *Logic. The theory of inquiry. The Later works of John Dewey*, vol. **12** (ed. J.A. Boyston). Carbondale & Edwardsville: Southern Illinois University Press.

General Medical Council (2020). *Guidance on Supporting Information for Appraisal and Revalidation.* London: GMC.

Chapter 7 **The Future of Medical Revalidation in the United Kingdom**

Introduction

The medical revalidation journey to this point has been, it could be argued, tortuous and arduous. The profession, the General Medical Council (GMC), with successive governments along with a range of key stakeholders such as the British Medical Association (BMA) and Royal Colleges, have all had to be dragged to the current position. It could be argued that the most influential set of factors that have acted as the sole catalysts for change were the numerous medical scandals that hit the press and shocked the public and patients, including the Bristol Royal Infirmary and the Paterson and Ayling cases. A recurrent theme with these cases was that individual doctors and others in the system at the time who were aware of the specific fitness-to-practice issues did not raise concerns. Even when concerns were raised, those charged with and having the authority to investigate the concerns and take appropriate action, if needed, did not do so. So what does the future hold for revalidation?

It would be prudent to revisit the initial aims of revalidation. The GMC and joint Chief Medical Officers (CMOs) from the four UK nations, in their statement in 2010, said:

> . . .*the purpose of revalidation is to assure patients and the public, employers and other health care professionals that licenced doctors are up to date and fit to practice.*

> (Pearson 2017)

In 2010, Peter Rubin, the Chair of the GMC at the time, declared that medical revalidation was the biggest change in regulation of doctors since 1858. So the key outcome of revalidation is to provide assurance that each doctor is

---

How to Succeed at Revalidation, First Edition. Peter Donnelly and Katie Webb.
© 2022 John Wiley & Sons Ltd. Published 2022 by John Wiley & Sons Ltd.

up to date and fit to practice. What evidence is there that it has achieved what it set out to do?

Despite the purpose of revalidation being stated clearly, there remains within the profession an almost delusional belief that the aims of revalidation are different than those stated above. As an example, Brown et al. (2020) states:

> *Appraisal has several objectives, including revalidation, performance management, and personal and professional development.*

The GMC has been very clear with regard to the purpose of appraisal and revalidation, emphasizing that it is not about performance management nor is it to identify and deal with serious concerns. There should be a range of other routes set within clinical governance processes for these concerns to be managed. If there are serious concerns, the Responsible Officer (RO) should not wait until the next revalidation to raise them, but is required via the RO regulations to instigate investigation locally and, if required, take appropriate action. This action may include referring the doctor to the GMC.

There have been a number of evaluations and reviews of revalidation. We have considered the Pearson Review (Pearson 2017) and the UK Medical Revalidation Evaluation coLLAboration (UMbRELLA) Report (2018) in Chapter 3. At the point of the Pearson Review, medical revalidation had been live for four years and a significant percentage of doctors had undergone their first revalidation. In his report, a wide range of data sources were used including data held by the GMC, any published work on the impact of revalidation, feedback from a range of organizations such as Royal Colleges, the BMA, NHS England and patient groups.

Pearson's conclusion was that appraisal and revalidation was taking place and that the principles underpinning it were essentially sound. His recommendations were aimed at tweaking the existing process as he concluded that the process was working well.

The UMbRELLA study, using a mixed methods approach, explored the regulatory impacts of revalidation between 2014 and 2017 (UMbRELLA 2018). This was a comprehensive study involving a range of approaches including undertaking nine literature reviews, surveying over 85 000 doctors, recording 44 appraisals, and interviews of 156 doctors and patient representatives. The key findings were that revalidation had been widely implemented but issues remained. These included uncertainty about the purpose and impact, higher deferral rates in black ethnic minority groups compared with white, and continuing confusion about what the full scope of practice entails.

The central finding was doctors reported that they had not changed their behavior as a result of appraisal. The authors argued that it was too early to assess cultural change like this, and further time was required for the processes to bed in.

In addition, there have been specific surveys of doctors to gather their views on the appraisal and revalidation process. These have provided inconclusive results. As one example, a survey undertaken by Health Education England (Cockman 2019) of over 13 000 GPs in a number of regions in England reported that over 90% of respondents stated that their appraisal was useful for promoting quality improvement in their work. In addition, 89% stated that they found it useful for improving patient care. This survey specifically asked about the experience of appraisal and not the wider process of revalidation. These very positive responses were in contrast with a survey undertaken by the Royal College of General Practitioners (RCGP) in 2017 where only 34% of GPs reported that appraisal promoted quality improvement (Royal College of General Practitioners 2018).

As suggested by the UMbRELLA study, the question remains; do we need longer to assess the impact of revalidation, to ensure that the aims and expected outcomes have been achieved on the basis that it takes time for culture to change?

But what is meant by the term culture? One useful definition of culture is:

> *The culture of a group can be defined as the accumulated shared learning of that group as it solves its problems of external adaption and internal integration; which has worked well enough to be considered valid and, therefore, to be taught to new members as the correct way to perceive, think, feel, and behave in relation to those problems.*

(Schein 2017, p. 6)

Another simpler definition is ". . .the way we do things around here" (Gray 2011, p. 144).

But one of the challenges in using this argument is that every doctor works at a different point in the complex adaptive system that is the NHS. The NHS is not one homogeneous organization. It is made up of thousands of subsystems each with their own subculture. In addition across the UK, since devolution of responsibility for health, the four systems have diverged significantly. This divergence encompasses the strategic model, delivery and funding models, structure, the role of competition, patient choice, and the use of non-NHS providers (Greer 2008).

So in the future will we see tinkering with the current system? There have been a number of alternative options put forward. These include:

- Enhanced appraisal
- Supporting information requiring validation
- External scrutiny of the appraisal process

- More direct involvement of patients and the public
- Moving closer to quality improvement as opposed to appraisal
- Online self-declarations
- Clinical audits
- Data signals from various sources
- A process of assessing competencies by direct observation.

But there are questions that need to be posed with regard to any assessment system. Using simple quality improvement methodology, these questions are:

- What is working well?
- What is not working so well?
- What can we learn from others in our own system?
- What can we learn from outside our system?
- How do we know it is working?

What current systems of assessment of fitness to practice exist in the medical system? What is the evidence that these systems are effective, that is, rigorously assess fitness to practice? Could these help steer any new direction of travel?

As far back as Liam Donaldson (Department of Health 2006), the option of assessing fitness to practice via direct observation in the real world and in simulated environments was considered and rejected on the basis of cost and the logistical problems in implementing it. But what is the cost of mistakes? This is not just the direct financial costs, but also the moral, ethical, personal and societal impact. In addition, what is the cost of further procrastination and delay for the profession as a whole, and more importantly for the public?

So what next? Is there a need for further changes? History suggests there will be. No one can predict the future, but history tells us that there will be societal pressure, and most likely increasingly so, to provide higher levels of assurance to the public that each doctor they see is up to date and fit to practice.

As a profession and as individuals working as doctors, is it appropriate to wait until there is another scandal, another BRI, another Mid Staffordshire, to then reluctantly accept that individual clinicians should be assessed on a regular basis?

What does the current system assess? It assesses whether a doctor has engaged with an annual appraisal process, as described in detail in Chapters 3 and 4. But what does that tell us? We argue it tests whether each doctor has engaged in the process. It does not in any way indicate any level of up-to-datedness with clinical knowledge nor fitness to practice.

The Argument against Direct Observation and Simulation Assessments

The arguments against any form of direct observation and simulation assessments are many, and include the following:

- Too expensive
- Logistically too difficult
- Unacceptable to the profession
- Unacceptable to medical trade unions, notably the BMA
- Unacceptable to the Royal Colleges
- Too challenging for the GMC to navigate the politics
- Too challenging for any government to navigate and/or survive the backlash from all of the above
- The process needs to be proportionate to the possible risks.

So will we be left with engagement in appraisal as a proxy for fitness to practice?

Some Resistances to Further Change

With the current medical revalidation process there are no assessments made of any individual doctor's competencies. Why is that? Is there a fear from individuals of failing assessments and the impact that might have on their ability to continue practicing? But that is the very purpose of revalidation, to assure fitness to practice. If any one individual is assessed as not fit to practice, then there will be a need to provide retraining or training and then reassessment. This process would meet the requirements of assurance: to provide the public with evidence of each doctor's fitness to practice. There was and is a feeling within the profession that is a step too far and could potentially have a significant impact on an individual and the health care system.

So what is the direction of travel? We have described the history of this journey in medicine and that all health and social professions are on the same trajectory. It has taken the UK and the medical profession from 1858 to 2012 to introduce some form of mandatory process.

Reflecting on the key findings from the UMbRELLA study, the conclusion was that the process needed further time to embed and effect change in doctors' behavior. What next, if further cycles of revalidation still do not lead to behavior change that improves quality of care for patients?

Does the current system provide assurance as it is supposed to? Assurance in its simplest terms is providing evidence of the desired outcome. So where is the evidence?

The GMC has a history of attempting to balance the needs of the public with political pressures and at the same time keeping their registrants happy. If the GMC decide that the best option is a system of direct observation of competencies, what reaction might there be? Will we see the BMA calling for strikes, withholding the licence fee en masse, as in 1976?

But the above reflections, we would argue, are missing the entire purpose of a regulator . . . that is to regulate. The GMC states on its website (GMC 2020):

> *We protect patients by making sure all doctors are registered with a licence to practise before they work in the UK.*

So how does appraisal protect patients? What is the evidence that the current process ensures a rigorous system that assesses all doctors' fitness to practice?

Is that what the current system does? As stated above, the only systematic review of medical revalidation in the UK (UMbRELLA 2018) showed a major issue, namely that doctors stated that their behavior has not changed.

The Conundrum

The definition of a conundrum is "a confusing and difficult problem or question." So the conundrum is that the current system is not designed to test fitness to practice. It is designed to test one's engagement in a non-validated annual appraisal.

Possible Solutions

The solution, or rather a set of solutions, currently exists in medicine. Before we offer these we wish to reflect on what we and most others consider to be a seminal review by Donaldson (Department of Health 2006).

This review was triggered by the Secretary of State for Health following the Fifth Shipman report in which Dame Janet Smith criticized the GMC's proposal to rely on annual appraisals of NHS doctors. She questioned whether this process would be a rigorous assessment of a doctor's performance. So at that point, the question remained as to whether annual appraisal cycles were an effective mechanism to identify doctors who were delivering poor quality of care or who were incompetent.

We wish to focus on this, as in our view the solutions have been described comprehensively but all dismissed at the time. Donaldson considered a number of high-risk industries and explored the regulatory processes in place at that time for civil aviation pilots, nuclear power unit desk engineers, and air traffic controllers. He described a number of common themes in these three high-risk industries. In the context of medical revalidation, one key theme was regular proficiency checks using direct observation and simulation.

Although acknowledging that these processes were rigorous, Donaldson argued that the transferability of these processes into medicine were not practical. He argued that as a result of the scale and number of doctors (at that time 170 000) compared with 17 000 pilots, the cost and logistics of using a similar process in medicine would not be feasible.

We will consider two key issues raised by Donaldson, the cost of a similar system in medicine and the comparison of risks.

Cost

The issue of cost at the time of the Donaldson report was a further argument against adopting similar regulatory processes to that of pilots. There would need to be an appropriate return on investment in any process. Since 2012 and the implementation of revalidation, the true direct recurring costs have been estimated at £100 million per year in England alone (White 2012).

What is the total cost of revalidation? Pearson reported that a positive outcome of medical revalidation was that it was locally owned. This raises the question of the direct additional costs of revalidation that every designated body has incurred to administer and monitor. These include:

- Appraisers' time
- Information technology systems (development and maintenance)
- Administrative and support staff
- Local appraisal teams
- Training for appraisers and appraisees
- Fees paid to General Practitioner appraisers
- Supporting Professional Activity time in hospital-based doctors' job plans.

What is the cost of medical negligence across the UK? Not all of this can be attributed to fitness to practice, but a proportion will be. In England, in the year 2018 to 2019 the value of claims rose by £6 billion from the previous year to a total of £83 billion, with the actual number of claims remaining level at approximately 10 600 (NHS Resolution 2019).

Comparison of Risks

Donaldson also stated that in these other high-risk industries, failure to perform can have a direct impact of the individual's safety and that of co-workers as well as the public. In medicine, however, the consequences of failure in performance of the doctor falls on a third party, the patient. The argument goes, if a pilot makes a mistake then the outcome could be the death of 250 humans. The fatality statistics for commercial aviation indicate that as a direct result of a number of systems including stringent training, retraining and direct observation of performance, that risk of death has reduced.

In 2019 the International Air Transport Association (IATA) released data for safety performance of the commercial airline industry across the world (International Air Transport Association 2019). This indicated continuing safety improvements over the long term in the aviation industry. The all-accident rate (measured in accidents per 1 million flights) was 1.35, the equivalent of one accident for every 740 000 flights. There were 11 fatal accidents resulting in 523 fatalities among passengers and crew.

A pilot making a mistake that doesn't result in a fatal crash will usually go unnoticed by the passengers. That is, in clinical language there is no morbidity or mortality as a result.

On the other hand, one doctor who is not fit to practice and as a result is making even minor mistakes can do significant damage to the long-term prognosis, morbidity and quality of life of hundreds, if not thousands, of patients. If one multiplies that across the UK with circa 335 000 doctors on the GMC register, what is the cost of not having a rigorous assessment of competency process similar, but not identical, to the commercial aviation industry?

Doctors are still in such a privileged and trusted position, but in general, even today, with clinical governance and national mortality audits such as in Cardiothoracic surgery (Bridgewater et al. 2013), it is still not inconceivable that another Paterson or Ayling event could happen.

Donaldson made a total of 44 recommendations, but the only ones directly related to the process of revalidation were (Department of Health 2006, p. xiv):

> *major changes to the structure, functions and governance of the General Medical Council;*
>
> *extension of the processes of medical regulation to the local level to create a stronger interface with the healthcare system;*
>
> *the creation of a clear, unambiguous and operationalized standard to define a good doctor, and its adoption into the contracts of all doctors;*
>
> *improved access for the public to timely and meaningful information about doctors, coupled with measures to ensure that such information is handled intelligently.*

Although it could be argued that most of these recommendations have been actioned, none of them directly addresses the issue of the implementation of a process to test fitness to practice.

Principles of a New System

We would suggest that a radical rethink of revalidation is needed – not a long protracted debate, but action to test other processes in identified test sites across the UK and across different specialties.

There are, in our view, a number of key principles that need to underpin any new, (not revised) system, and these are:
- Testing an individual doctor's fitness to practice
- The process being independent from, but linked to the employer
- Clear standards published against which each doctor will be assessed
- A process of appeal against serious fitness to practice issues
- A graded approach to the assessment
- Access to timely and appropriate training
- Any constraints in the system need to be to be taken into consideration.

These and other checks and balances are required, in particular to safeguard doctors and to ensure the processes are transparent and mitigate the risk of inappropriate assessments that may affect a doctor's ability to continue practicing and/or damage their reputation.

A New Model

Reflecting back on one of the key quality improvement questions: what can we learn from systems already operational in the UK's health care system that have been tried and tested?

Doctors in formal training programs across the UK are subject to a high number of regular assessments, including direct observation of procedures, analysis of recordings of consultations, and case-based discussion. Doctors in training are required to show progress against each of these mapped to the requirements in the GMC approved curricula. In effect the trainee is required to "pass" to enable them to progress in their training. Therefore, there is a system already in existence that, although not without its critics, has been tried and tested on over 60 000 doctors in training per annum since the introduction of Modernizing Medical Careers in 2005.

Using the current assessment blueprint for those doctors in training with a National Training Number (NTN), there is a clear movement to add in not just assessment of procedures, but a broader and higher level concept of capabilities. As an example, the new General Internal Medicine (GIM) curriculum introduced in the UK in 2018 provides a useful model. In the context of GIM this is the difference between "Can I insert a chest drain?" and "Can I run an acute medical assessment unit?"

The purpose of the assessment process for GIM as stated on the Joint Royal Colleges of Physicians Training Board (JRCPTB) website includes the following:

> *provide robust, summative evidence that trainees are meeting the curriculum standards during the training programme;*
> *ensure trainees are acquiring competencies within the domains of Good Medical Practice;*
> *assess trainees' actual performance in the workplace;*
> *ensure that trainees possess the essential underlying knowledge required for their specialty.*
>
> (Joint Royal Colleges of Physicians Training Board 2021)

The assessment system for GIM is similar to all other assessment schedules across the postgraduate curricula in the UK. This comprises a mixture of workplace-based assessments (WPBAs) and knowledge-based assessments. Within training programs the WPBAs take place continually throughout the annual cycle.

The assessments in GIM that use direct observation of performance are:

1 **Mini-Clinical Evaluation Exercise (mini-CEX)**

   Mini-Clinical Evaluation Exercise (mini-CEX) is a directly supervised learning event (SLE) tool widely used across most postgraduate curricula in the UK. The supervisor directly observes the doctor-in-training's clinical encounter with a patient and provides immediate feedback on a range of areas, including history-taking, physical examination, communication, diagnostic skills, and clinical decision-making. Mini-CEXs can be used flexibly in any clinical setting as a learning opportunity.

2 **Direct Observation of Procedural Skills (DOPS)**

   A Direct Observation of Procedural Skills (DOPS) is an assessment tool designed to assess the performance in undertaking a specific practical procedure. The supervisor assesses the doctor against an agreed structured checklist. Formative DOPS allow the doctor in training to receive feedback and improve their performance under direct supervision. At certain points a summative DOPS will be undertaken.

3 **Acute Care Assessment Tool (ACAT)**

   The Acute Care Assessment Tool (ACAT) is designed to assess the doctor-in-training's capability to perform a range of tasks on an acute medical take. This is a broader assessment of their ability to manage and lead the acute take.

These assessments are in addition to case-based discussions, patient surveys, audits, multi-source feedback (MSF) and observation of teaching. So within the training programs, direct observation of the doctor-in-training is a routine and frequently used tool to assess competencies in clinical and non-clinical settings.

We are proposing that a region in the UK should be identified to test the new process. It is imperative the test sites are adequately supported and resourced with the aim of assessing whether the process is fit for purpose (i.e. to assess a doctor's fitness to practice).

Adopting some of the tools used in the commercial aviation industry, an independent assessor may arrive unannounced at out-patients, in theaters and in Multi-Disciplinary Teams. Are doctors so special that this would be unacceptable? We are now in the twenty-first century, and we would argue it has taken centuries to get to mandatory appraisal. What does that say about medicine as a profession?

We would suggest that a pilot is focused on high-risk procedures, high-impact interventions decided upon by the data, currently available in the system.

Process to Oversee New Model

Any new process will require independent external governance arrangements. This could take the form of an independent medical revalidation office on a regional basis.

As mentioned above, there is already a significant amount of resources dedicated to appraisal and revalidation across all health care systems in the UK. No doubt implementing an independent process to assess doctors directly in real time will incur additional direct cost, but there would be an opportunity to redeploy staff currently supporting all the requirements of a formal mandatory appraisal. Additional funding will be required, but a key aim of the pilot would be to evaluate the cost–benefit ratio to measure value for money.

As an initial step, direct observation assessments could focus on specific high-risk, high competence procedures driven by the datasets already available.

What about the voice of the patients, those who have been subject to the care provided by a doctor? Are they not best placed to provide evidence? The patient-reported outcome measures and patient-reported experience measures have only been introduced and embedded sporadically in the UK. The concept of the active patient is recognized (Hibbard and Gilburt 2014), but again, not embedded in a systematic way.

Chapter Summary

The biggest change in the regulation of doctors in the 163 years since 1858 has been the introduction of mandatory annual appraisal. The supporting information used by individual doctors that is central to this process is not validated. Engagement with five annual appraisals with at least one MSF from patients (in that five-year cycle) entitles a doctor to maintain their license to practice. Is this really acceptable in the twenty-first century?

Other high-risk professions have invested in direct observation of fitness to practice along with the use of simulation assessments. The direct observations in the case of commercial pilots is in real time: the "capabilities," in medical training language. These professions have invested so that the public can be assured, and to a certain extent reassured, that the risk is minimized. The role of any doctor carries with it a level of risk, and we argue that needs to be accepted by the profession and individual doctors themselves. We argue for the testing of a process that isn't novel, as it has been used in formal medical training programs across the UK since the introduction of Modernizing Medical Careers in 2005. This entails direct observation of doctors working in real time with patients, interacting with health colleagues and other staff. These DOPs can be planned and unplanned. There needs to be a no-blame culture for this to work. Does that exist? Probably not, but it is improving slowly. A culture needs to develop where any gaps in skills or knowledge are not an indication of failure but just signals the need for further targeted continuing professional development.

How is the public currently assured of the fitness to practice of every doctor in the UK? Essentially the public have to trust the GMC and employers to oversee a process that assesses each doctor. How publicly transparent is that process? The RO will see the summary of any appraisal so that it can be sense-checked, which basically means that there is a statement to say there are no concerns raised and the doctor is engaged in the appraisal process. Any member of the public can access the GMC medical register to check the status of any doctor. That status is that the doctor is engaged in annual appraisal. It is a challenge to understand how this process provides transparency.

The status of the medical profession in society has been eroded in recent years. The implicit social contract has become more explicit, with an evolving change in the power balance between doctors and their patients. Patients come to the doctor with more information and understanding gathered from the internet. Patients and their relatives are now, correctly, more aware of their rights.

The journey from the days when doctors underwent training and were signed off as "the expert," be that a GP or consultant, the so-called autonomous clinician with no further assessment of their fitness to undertake even basic interventions is unacceptable. The journey from nothing to mandatory appraisal has taken many years. As a profession, can doctors sit quietly, or not so quietly, resisting further change to provide the public they serve with assurance that each is fit to practice?

References

Bridgewater, B., Hickey, G.L., Cooper, G. et al. (2013). Publishing cardiac surgery mortality rates: lessons for other specialties. *British Medical Journal* **346**: f1139. https://doi.org/10.1136/bmj.f1139.

Brown, V.T., McCartney, M., and Heneghan, C. (2020). Appraisal and revalidation for UK doctors – time to assess the evidence. *British Medical Journal* **19**: 361–363.

Cockman, P. (2019). *Medical appraisal: Feedback from GPs in 2018–19*. NHS England and NHS Improvement. https://www.england.nhs.uk/wp-content/uploads/2019/07/medical-appraisal-feedback-from-gps-18-19-v1.1.pdf (accessed 21 May 2021).

Department of Health (2006). Good doctors, safer patients. Proposals to strengthen the system to assure and improve the performance of doctors and to protect the safety of patients. A report by the Chief Medical Officer. London: Department of Health. https://webarchive.nationalarchives.gov.uk/20080728114331/http://www.dh.gov.uk/en/Publicationsandstatistics/Publications/PublicationsPolicyAndGuidance/DH_4137232 (accessed 7 May 2021).

General Medical Council (2020). Registration and licensing. https://www.gmc-uk.org/registration-and-licensing (accessed 20 May 2021).

Gray, J.A.M. (2011). *How to Build Health Care Systems*. Offox Press for Better Healthcare Ltd.

Greer, S.L. (2008). Devolution and divergence in UK health policies. *British Medical Journal* **337** https://doi.org/10.1136/bmj.a2616.

Hibbard, J. and Gilburt, H. (2014). *Supporting People to Manage their Health. An Introduction to Patient Activation*. London: The King's Fund.

International Air Transport Association (2019) IATA Releases 2018 Airline Safety Performance. https://www.iata.org/en/pressroom/pr/2019-02-21-01/ (accessed 21 May 2021).

Joint Royal Colleges of Physicians Training Board (2021). *Workplace based assessment.* https://www.jrcptb.org.uk/assessment/workplace-based-assessment (accessed 21 May).

NHS Resolution (2019). Clinical negligence numbers steady, but rising costs remain a concern. https://resolution.nhs.uk/2019/07/11/clinical-negligence-numbers-steady-but-rising-costs-remain-a-concern/ (accessed 21 May 2021).

Pearson, K. (2017). *Taking revalidation forward. Improving the process of relicensing for doctors*. Manchester: General Medical Council. https://www.gmc-uk.org/-/media/documents/Taking_revalidation_forward___Improving_the_process_of_relicensing_for_doctors.pdf_68683704.pdf (accessed 5 May 2021).

Royal College of General Practitioners (2018). *RCGP Revalidation Survey, 2017. Key findings and conclusions.* London: RCGP Revalidation Survey. https://www.rcgp.org.uk/-/media/Files/Revalidation-and-CPD/2018/RCGP-revalidation-survey-report-2017.ashx?la=en (accessed 21 May 2021).

Schein, E.H. (2017). *Organization Culture and Leadership*, 5e. Jossey-Bass.

UK Medical Revalidation coLLAboration (2018). *Evaluating the regulatory impact of medical revalidation.* https://www.gmc-uk.org/-/media/documents/umbrella-report-final_pdf-74454378.pdf (accessed 8 May 2021).

White, C. (2012). Revalidation will cost nearly £100m a year. *British Medical Journal* **345**: e7659.

Index

Page locators in **bold** indicate tables. Page locators in *italics* indicate figures. This index uses letter-by-letter alphabetization.

How to Succeed at Revalidation, First Edition. Peter Donnelly and Katie Webb.
© 2022 John Wiley & Sons Ltd. Published 2022 by John Wiley & Sons Ltd.